OKINAWA KATA ENCYCLOPEDIA

OKINAWA KATA ENCYCLOPEDIA

EXPLORING RYUKYU'S MARTIAL SECRETS

Nathan Batson

Guardian Arts Press, Murchison, TX

Published by Guardian Arts Press

Murchison, Texas

Book Cover design and photography by BatCave Studios

ISBN: 979-8-9924113-2-4

Library of Congress Control Number: 2025920695

Printed in the United States of America

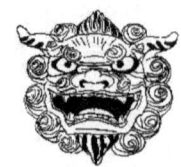

Guardian Arts Press

In memory of Isao Kise — master, mentor, and friend.

Though his passing in February 2025 left a silence beyond words, his legacy endures in every kata, every lesson I teach, and every student who carries his art forward.

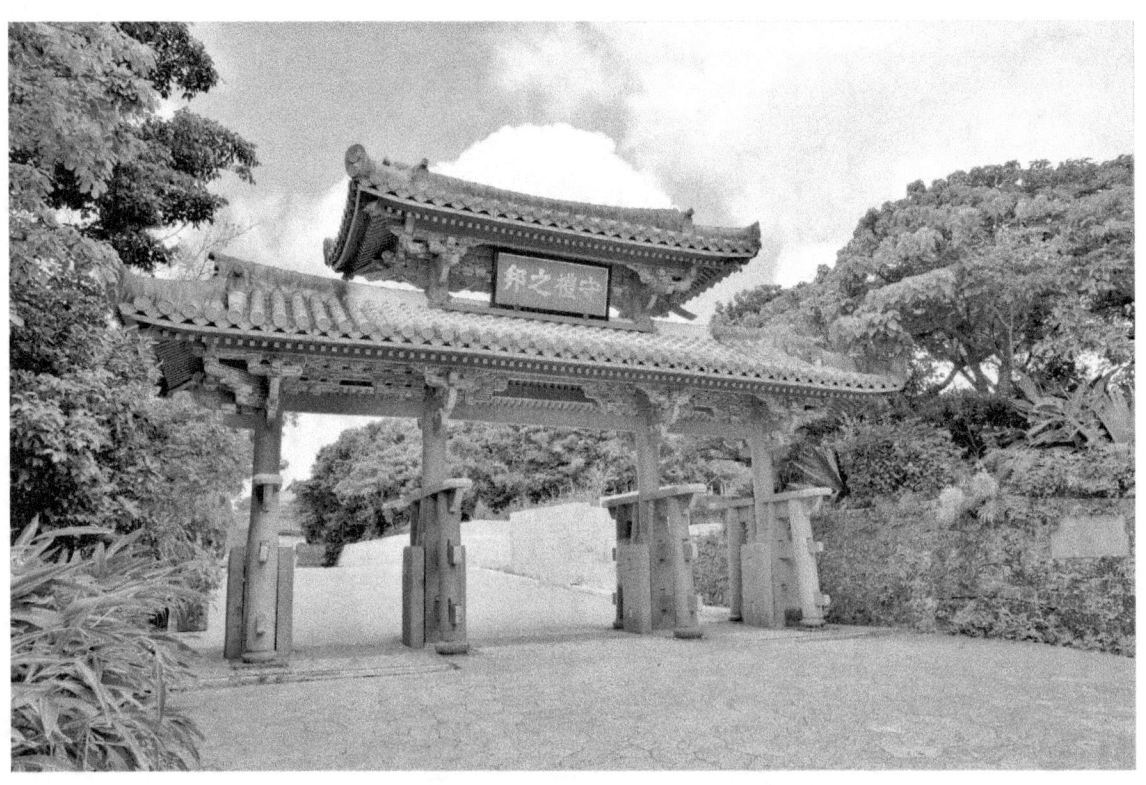

Shureimon Gate, Shuri Castle (守礼門). The famous "Gate of Courtesy," welcoming visitors to the royal palace complex.

(October 2010)

PREFACE

This work originated from a simple observation: while many excellent books on karate and kobudō exist, I have not found a single volume that comprehensively gathers the full range of kata in a way that is both accessible and respectful of tradition. I believed it would be helpful to create a reference that offers concise overviews of individual kata, discussing their origins, historical contexts, and interpretations across different lineages. My hope is that both practitioners and enthusiasts will find this resource valuable, enabling them to appreciate not only the kata of their own school but also those practiced by others.

This book does not claim to unveil anything groundbreaking or revolutionary. Instead, it serves as a collection, an encyclopedia in the truest sense, of explanations, insights, and perspectives that have been passed down, studied, and debated over time. Its purpose is not to dictate a single "truth," but to provide readers with a framework for deeper study and comparison, and perhaps to spark new questions about the forms they practice.

If this work succeeds, it will serve as a companion: a resource to consult, reflect upon, and return to over time, as one's own journey through kata continues to evolve.

ACKNOWLEDGMENTS

This work could not have been completed without the guidance and inspiration of the late Kise Isao, former Kaicho of the OSMKKF and heir to Matsumura Seito Karate and Kobudō, as well as my teacher, John Shipes Hanshi. Their mentorship has profoundly shaped both my practice and perspective, and I remain deeply grateful for their example.

I also want to express my gratitude to the many practitioners who have shared their knowledge through research, writing, and video. Their efforts have allowed me to gain deeper insights, truly standing, as Isaac Newton wrote, "on the shoulders of giants." The support from my peers in the OSMKKF and the students of Tyler Karate Academy has further grounded this project, providing invaluable feedback, encouragement, and a living reminder of the vitality of kata.

Lastly, I acknowledge all those across different systems and styles who have contributed to the preservation and transmission of Okinawan martial traditions. This book serves, in part, as a testament to their collective efforts and to the enduring spirit of kata itself.

INTRODUCTION

Kata are simultaneously simple and complex. To the untrained eye, they may seem like choreographed movements; an elaborate dance of stances, strikes, and steps. However, to the practitioner, kata are much more than mere sequences; they serve as repositories of principles, strategies, and philosophies. Each form encodes not only combat techniques but also lessons in rhythm, timing, breathing, and character development. They are cultural artifacts as well as martial exercises, bridging centuries of Okinawan experience.

The kata of Okinawa emerged within a unique historical context. The Ryukyu Kingdom, located at the crossroads of East Asia, was shaped by exchanges with Chinese tributary systems, indigenous fighting traditions, and the realities of Satsuma occupation. Over time, these influences melded into the practices we now recognize as karate and kobudō. Kata became the means by which knowledge was preserved and transmitted, refined by each generation of teachers and adapted to meet the needs of their students. Some forms traveled widely and evolved into various versions, while others remained closely guarded within specific lineages.

This encyclopedia aims to explore both the familiar and the obscure. From foundational empty-hand kata like Sanchin and Pinan to weapon forms such as Chatan Yara no Sai and Tsuken Sunakake no Eku, each chapter offers a concise overview of the kata's origins, naming, historical context, and major interpretations. When there is certainty in history, it is noted; when traditions diverge, multiple perspectives are presented. The intention is not to provide definitive answers but to help readers appreciate the depth of their own practice and the broader web of Okinawan martial culture.

The structure of the encyclopedia progresses from beginner to advanced kata and from empty-hand forms to kobudō. Each entry follows a consistent format: introduction, name breakdown, historical roots, combat applications, evolving traditions, and lasting impact. This organization allows readers to trace not only the technical features of a kata but also its cultural and historical significance.

Kata are neither sacred relics nor empty motions. They represent structured, significant, and evolving links to the past that continue to influence the practice of martial artists today. It is in this spirit that this encyclopedia has been compiled: as a reference, a companion, and an invitation to delve more deeply into the traditions we inherit.

TABLE OF CONTENTS

BOOK ONE - KARATE
DECODING THE EMPTY HAND

Kata has been a foundational element in Okinawan martial arts for generations, yet it remains a topic of debate. Some practitioners view it as a living manuscript of ancient combat techniques, while others see it as a stylized relic; performed without proper understanding and displayed without critical examination. This work does not fully embrace either perspective. Kata is neither sacred nor meaningless; it is structured, significant, and evolving. When approached critically and physically, it serves as a uniquely effective means of transmitting principles across time.

This volume does not aim to glorify kata nor to simplify it into mere performance. Instead, the goal is to explore each form as a convergence of history, culture, and combat wisdom. What are its origins? What does its name truly imply? What influences have guided its development? What mechanics and strategic concepts does it embody? These questions are not tangential; they are essential, particularly for those seeking to move beyond mere repetition to a functional understanding.

The first half of this work concentrates solely on the empty-hand kata of Okinawan karate. I have categorized them into three groups: foundational kata that establish the groundwork, intermediate kata that build upon that foundation, and advanced kata that delve into various schools of thought based on principles from earlier forms. While some might dispute this classification due to the specific focus of their own style or school, I have aimed to adopt a broader perspective regarding how kata is generally understood in the context of Okinawan karate. Each chapter is organized not by rank or difficulty but as individual case studies, treating each as a self-contained system of knowledge while ensuring thematic balance and historical contrast. This structure allows for meaningful comparisons between forms that share principles or diverge in interesting ways.

The writing is methodical, but not mechanical. Every chapter follows a consistent structure: Exploring Kata's Essence, origins and development, technical and internal principles, applications, evolution, and lasting significance. Notable historical figures are discussed, and persistent myths are examined rather than simply repeated.

Readers should approach this text with an understanding that certainty is often elusive. In many cases, historical records are scant, oral traditions conflict, and interpretations vary by school or agenda. This aspect is integral to kata's legacy: it has endured through adaptation, reinterpretation, and a resistance to oversimplification. However, there is a distinction between a system that evolves and one that simply drifts. This book aims to clarify that distinction by revealing the layered logic behind each kata's design, movement, and preservation.

Kata has long been described as a method for transmitting combat knowledge when practice needed to be concealed or condensed. This may hold true, but kata also conveys something more profound: a way of moving, a way of perceiving, and a way of embodying a martial heritage that transcends the battlefield. This book is intended for practitioners and instructors who seek a comprehensive collection of information and are eager to deepen their understanding of kata and its significance within the rich tradition of Okinawan karate. If this book succeeds, it will not be because it answers every historical question, but because it encourages readers to ask better ones.

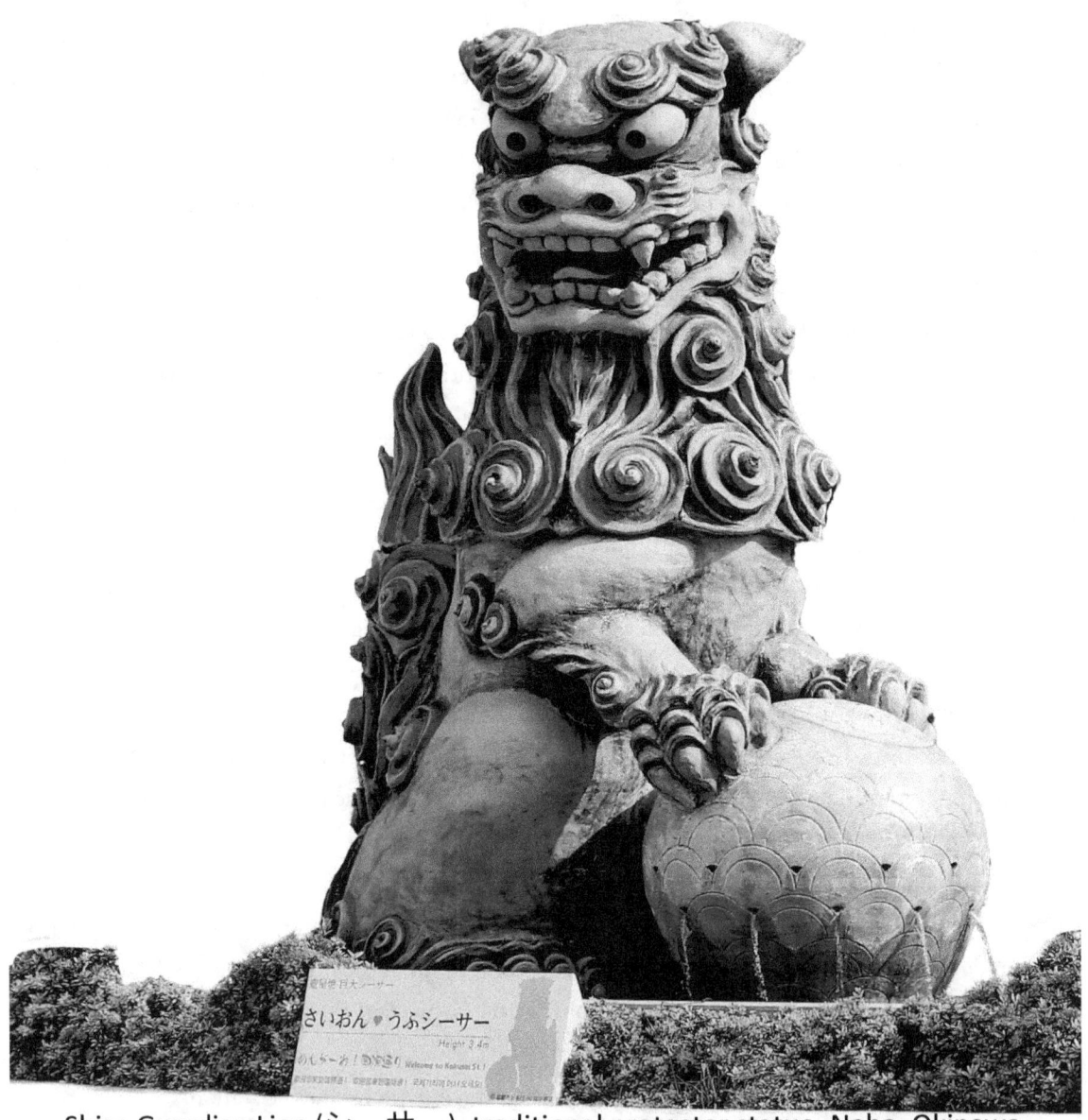

Shisa Guardian Lion (シーサー), traditional protector statue, Naha, Okinawa.

(July 2019)

SECTION I - FOUNDATIONAL KATA

OKINAWA'S FOUNDATIONS:
"FORGING THE CORE: OKINAWA'S MARTIAL BEGINNINGS"

"Foundational" kata are often misunderstood. To the untrained eye or the impatient student, they can seem rudimentary. Their techniques are straightforward, their patterns repetitive, and their footwork appears static. However, within these early forms lies a rich depth of structure that requires years to fully understand. These kata are not merely for beginners; they serve as the foundational practice for experts.

In Okinawan martial systems, foundational forms serve multiple purposes: they teach posture and positioning, introduce the principles of balance and breath, and establish the body mechanics upon which all subsequent material is built. In many lineages, these kata are also used to assess whether practitioners have internalized essential skills, such as generating power from the ground, maintaining tension and release, and expressing intention through rhythm. These are not skills to be graduated from; rather, they are skills to be revisited and refined over time.

This section includes both modern instructional kata, like the Fukyugata and Pinan series, which were created to standardize and simplify early training, as well as much older core forms such as Naihanchi, Seisan, and Sanchin, which were historically taught privately or preserved within family lineages. The modern forms are designed with teaching in mind, while the older forms have survived because they encode valuable principles worth preserving. Together, they represent not a sequential curriculum, but a set of conceptual foundations that anchor the practitioner's body, breath, and strategy from the very beginning.

SANCHIN
OKINAWA'S THREE BATTLES

INTRODUCTION TO SANCHIN

At first glance, Sanchin may seem deceptively simple. It lacks sweeping kicks, spinning strikes, or acrobatic movements, relying instead on rooted stances, controlled breathing, and deliberate steps. However, for those who train in it seriously, Sanchin serves as a crucible—a kata that facilitates transformation rather than mere spectacle. The challenges it presents are internal, and its refinements are lifelong.

As the foundational kata of Naha-te, Sanchin is a cornerstone for styles like Goju-ryu, Uechi-ryu, and Shito-ryu. It is specifically designed to cultivate internal strength, correct posture, controlled breathing, and unwavering mental focus. Sanchin functions as a method for body conditioning, a meditative practice, and a combat-oriented training drill, with its principles deeply rooted in Southern Chinese martial arts.

In the following sections, we will explore the layered complexity of Sanchin. We will trace its origins from Southern China to Okinawa, examine the evolution of its structure, unpack its internal mechanics, and analyze its significant role as both a physical and philosophical foundation. Sanchin is not just an introductory kata; it serves as a continuous mirror for the martial artist's development.

EXPLORING SANCHIN'S ESSENCE

- **Traditional Notation**: 三戦 (Sanchin); also サンチン in some texts.
- **Script Breakdown**:
    - 三 "three";
    - 戦 "battle/struggle."
- **Core Meaning**: "Three Battles" (body–mind–breath or three lines of power).
- **Modern Interpretations**: Goju/Uechi often frame the "three" as internal integrations; some read it as three stages of training.
- **Conflicting Ideas & Origins**: Name itself is stable; debate centers on what the "three" denotes (no strong alternate kanji traditions).

The term Sanchin (三戦), which translates to "Three Battles," has multiple meanings that contribute to its significant importance. Unlike many other kata, which are often referred to by their names in katakana, Sanchin has consistently been recognized by its kanji. This distinction highlights its foundational role within the martial traditions of Okinawa. The name itself comprises the characters 三 (San) meaning "three," and 戦 (Chin) denoting "battle" or "war." This name is not linked to a specific geographic origin or individual; rather, it embodies a universal concept: the internal struggle for self-mastery.

One prevalent interpretation of Sanchin emphasizes the unification of three essential elements that must be mastered: mind, body, and spirit. In the context of Buddhism, Sanchin can also symbolize the three enemies that must be overcome on the path to enlightenment: greed, anger, and ignorance. Additionally, the kata's specific breathing techniques are believed to have physical benefits, such as strengthening the lungs, heart, and kidneys. These interpretations collectively emphasize the holistic nature of Sanchin, which encompasses not only physical training but also a deeper philosophical journey toward balance and self-mastery. In both Okinawan and Chinese traditions, the number three often symbolizes harmony, making "Three Battles" a fitting metaphor for the lifelong internal process that lies at the heart of budo.

SANCHIN'S HISTORICAL ORIGINS

A fundamental aspect of the Naha-te tradition, Sanchin acts as an important link between Chinese and Okinawan martial arts. Its origins are rooted in the mid-to-late Qing dynasty period of 19th-century China, though its influences likely extend even further back to traditions of Chinese Buddhist temple boxing, qigong practices, and the Fujian White Crane systems. This strong connection to Southern Chinese martial arts is evident in its structure, which heavily incorporates elements from traditions such as Southern Shaolin Qigong and Monk Fist Boxing.

Sanchin's introduction to Okinawa is credited to Higaonna Kanryo, who traveled to Fuzhou, China, to study various Kung Fu styles under masters like RuRuKo. Upon returning to Okinawa in the late 19th century, Higaonna began teaching the techniques he had learned in China, adapting the Sanchin kata to fit the local context, establishing his own dojo and incorporating rigorous physical and mental training.

The Sanchin he taught was different from the Chinese version; he made several key modifications, including slowing the breathing and techniques to highlight their conditioning and health benefits. This adaptation was crucial as karate started to be introduced to schoolchildren, necessitating a focus on physical fitness. Additionally, he famously introduced the closed fist, in contrast to the open spear hand typically used in the Chinese version.

Ultimately, the main purpose of Sanchin goes beyond being just a performance kata. It is primarily a forging practice intended to develop internal strength and a solid physical structure while conditioning the body to withstand impact. It also serves as a framework for breath control through techniques like ibuki. Through dedicated practice, Sanchin significantly influences the practitioner's form, function, and mental focus, making it a powerful tool for transformation rather than merely a series of movements. It is also believed to be related to a broader family of forms that includes Sanseru, Seipai, and Suparinpei.

APPLYING SANCHIN'S COMBAT WISDOM

While it may appear to have minimal surface movements, Sanchin encompasses a rich variety of key techniques and applications. The core movements of the kata subtly integrate elbow strikes, short punches, and blocks that also function as limb traps. In some versions, palm heel strikes are included as well. The practice emphasizes fundamental grappling techniques, underscoring the importance of disrupting an opponent's root and maintaining control through contact.

These techniques are not just theoretical; they are practical applications for close-range combat. They prepare practitioners to intercept attacks, bridge gaps, and manage space effectively within clinch range. Consequently, the bunkai, or applications, are often taught separately, requiring a high level of tactile sensitivity to develop the quick reactions and adaptability needed in high-pressure situations.

Additionally, Sanchin serves as a foundational training method within Okinawan karate, shaping both the practitioner's body and mind through focused principles. It incorporates ibuki, an audible diaphragmatic breathing technique that synchronizes movement and breath. Practitioners also cultivate kime, which emphasizes muscle contraction during movement to maximize power, and muchimi, a "sticky" or heavy body feel achieved through a precise balance of tension and timing. Finally, a key element is chinkuchi, which involves the instantaneous locking of joints to generate powerful short-range energy, thereby enhancing the effectiveness of strikes and techniques executed in close proximity.

SANCHIN'S DIVERSE PATHS

A foundational practice in various karate styles, with a rich transmission history, Sanchin was originally passed down from the renowned martial artist Higaonna to several key figures. Among these figures were Miyagi Chojun, who played a significant role in Goju-ryu; Mabuni Kenwa, the founder of Shito-ryu; and Uechi Kanbun, who established Uechi-ryu. Each of these martial artists incorporated Sanchin into their teachings, adding their own distinct nuances. Additionally, the Matayoshi family and other lesser-known systems also adopted Sanchin, demonstrating its versatility.

The stylistic variations of Sanchin are noteworthy. In Goju-ryu, practitioners use closed fists, maintain a static form without turning, and utilize loud ibuki breathing to enhance their practice. In contrast, while Shito-ryu retains similarities to Goju-ryu, it often features a softer approach to breathing. Uechi-ryu stands out by using open-handed techniques and placing a slightly different structural emphasis on the execution of Sanchin. This distinction is believed by many to stem from Uechi Kanbun's unique interpretation brought over from China. The Matayoshi system further enriches Sanchin by including multiple kata, such as Shuri Sanchin and Tsuru Sanchin.

The variations within Sanchin can be attributed to several key factors. Individual practitioners, including Chojun Miyagi, the founder of Goju-ryu, have made personal modifications to kata based on their unique experiences and understanding. These adjustments reflect their insights into balance, tension, and breathing techniques that enhance practice. Different styles of karate place varying degrees of emphasis on underlying internal systems, body mechanics, and breath control, catering to distinct teaching methodologies for both beginners and advanced students.

For instance, some schools may prioritize the martial application and practical self-defense elements of Sanchin, while others focus on the meditative and holistic aspects, encouraging a deeper connection between mind and body. Additionally, adaptations to Sanchin have been made to accommodate diverse body types, recognizing that physical differences can influence how the kata is executed. Overall, these factors contribute to a rich tapestry of interpretations and practices within the kata.

As a result, Sanchin serves as a foundational element not only within its own system but also across other forms of martial arts; its principles evident in kata such as Tensho and Sanseru. The stances and breathing techniques developed in Sanchin have also influenced the foundational training practices of many other martial arts.

SANCHIN'S LASTING IMPACT

Sanchin is much more than just a simple kata; it serves as a foundational crucible for everything that comes after it. Its seemingly limited movements hide layers of profound depth, ranging from internal mechanics and breath control to the development of a strong power structure, mental discipline, and subtle applications. With roots tracing back to Southern China and evolving in Okinawa, Sanchin embodies both the beginning and essence of martial refinement.

More than just a kata of physical motion, Sanchin represents a lifelong practice. Its foundational principles continuously resurface in advanced kata, applied techniques, and the composed demeanor of experienced practitioners. To study Sanchin is, in essence, to study oneself. The Three Battles, of body, breath, and mind, are never fully conquered but are faced each day with increasing clarity and resolve.

NAIHANCHI
OKINAWA'S IRON ROOTS

INTRODUCTION TO NAIHANCHI

At first glance, Naihanchi may appear deceptively simple; its lateral stepping, rooted horse stance, and linear movements might seem limited in range and application, but beneath its dry exterior lies a kata of remarkable depth, revered by many Okinawan masters as fundamental to true martial understanding. Chojun Miyagi once described it as the most critical kata for developing foundational power, while Nagamine Shoshin regarded it as a primer for body mechanics. Its lineage traces back to legendary figures such as Matsumura Sokon and Itosu Anko, and its variations reflect the diversity of Okinawa's fighting systems.

This chapter explores the contested history, core techniques, and ongoing evolution of Naihanchi. We examine its disputed Chinese origins, analyze its bunkai and biomechanical principles, and compare how different styles have interpreted and preserved this crucial form.

EXPLORING NAIHANCHI'S ESSENCE

- **Traditional Notation:** ナイハンチ/ナイファンチ; also 内歩進; historic orthography is unsettled.
- **Script Breakdown:**
    - 内 "inside";
    - 歩 "step";
    - 進 "advance."
    - Together (proposed): "advance with internal/side steps."
- **Core Meaning:** Commonly glossed as "internal/side stepping" kata (fits its lateral embusen).
- **Modern Interpretations:** Shotokan renames the series "Tekki" (鉄騎 "iron horse"), emphasizing the stance over the obscure toponym.
- **Conflicting Ideas & Origins:**
    - Competing folk etymologies (place names, Chinese readings).
    - No conclusive primary source for original kanji; most scholars treat 内歩進 as a plausible back-formation.

The kata known as Naihanchi (or Naifanchi) has long been a subject of considerable debate among martial arts practitioners regarding the true meaning of its name. While some interpret it as "sideward fighting" due to its distinctive lateral movement, others contend its origins lie in a Southern Chinese form called Naihanchin.

When looking at the name for clues, it is crucial to note that the earliest written references to this kata primarily list it only in Katakana (ナイハンチ). This linguistic choice is highly significant because Katakana in Japanese is typically reserved for loanwords from other languages or for emphasis, suggesting "Naihanchi" was considered a foreign or non-standard Japanese term at the time. Given this, the various kanji interpretations applied by modern practitioners – such as breaking down "nai" as "inside," "han" as "barrier," and "chi" (or "te") as "hand" to suggest close-quarters combat in confined spaces – are likely later, speculative adaptations rather than reflections of the kata's original, lost meaning. Despite their speculative nature, these interpretations are often cited to highlight the kata's focus on stability, immovability, and forward pressure, and may even metaphorically suggest internal confrontation or the perseverance needed to overcome obstacles. However, it is important to remember that such kanji associations lack direct historical evidence from the earliest records.

Naihanchi's Historical Origins

The Naihanchi kata has deep roots in Okinawan martial arts, with evidence suggesting that its core principles and techniques might even predate the 1609 Satsuma invasion. This connection is supported by historical ties to Chinese martial arts, the longstanding trade and cultural exchange between China and Okinawa, and the existence of native Okinawan fighting traditions prior to the occupation.

One of the oldest known references to the kata comes from Motobu Choki, who explicitly stated that Naihanchi was imported from China but was no longer practiced there during his time. Therefore, it is likely that Naihanchi, at the very least, emerged during the 18th and 19th centuries as a foundational component of the evolving Shuri-te tradition.

Matsumura Sokon (circa 1809–1899) is often credited with introducing Naihanchi to Okinawa. Its status and form were further developed by Itosu Anko (1831–1915), who expanded the kata into three distinct parts: Naihanchi Shodan, Nidan, and Sandan. Itosu's significant public school reforms and his efforts to standardize karate instruction greatly enhanced the importance of Naihanchi, establishing it as a fundamental kata for beginners.

In the early days of modern karate training, students commonly spent two to three intense years practicing nothing but Naihanchi under strict guidance from their teachers. This rigorous focus highlights the kata's profound depth. Designed specifically for practical close-range fighting, Naihanchi is highly effective in developing essential attributes such as lateral strength, rooting, and integrated upper-body mechanics. Its deceptive simplicity hides a sophisticated emphasis on structure, pressure application, and efficient, powerful movement. For Itosu, it served as an accessible form to help students build foundational skills; for Matsumura, it embodied the raw realism crucial for combat effectiveness. By the Meiji era, Itosu's reforms had firmly established Naihanchi at the forefront of karate instruction.

APPLYING NAIHANCHI'S COMBAT WISDOM

The foundational kata, Naihanchi (also known as Tekki in some styles), serves as a cornerstone of Karate instruction and is recognized for its unique Naihanchi dachi stance. However, the execution of this stance varies greatly across different karate styles and lineages, particularly regarding the direction of the toes. These variations, whether the toes point inward, outward, or straight forward, each have distinct reasons and interpretations, reflecting the kata's evolution and the various emphases within different traditions.

When the toes point inward (often referred to as Naihanchi Dachi or Gyaku-hachiji-dachi), some lineages believe that this configuration, typically with aligned knees and hips, maximizes rotational power from the legs and hips. This stance enables the generation of significant force in close-range combat without extensive movement while also providing a strong internal structure that protects the groin and midsection. The narrower, toes-in stance is considered highly effective in confined spaces.

Conversely, when the toes point outward (as in Shiko Dachi or Sumo Stance), the stance gains exceptional stability against forward pressure, similar to sumo wrestling. This configuration allows for effectively projecting force in a specific direction, akin to certain applications in Taijiquan. It tends to be a deeper, lower stance, which is advantageous for grappling but may sacrifice some mobility.

Many schools, including some Shotokan and Shito-ryu lineages, utilize Kiba Dachi (Horse Stance), where the feet are parallel and point straight forward. This traditional interpretation promotes rapid sideways movement and aligns with the kata's linear, side-to-side transitions. It also provides a structure for grounding against force from multiple directions without the specific rotational focus of the toes-in variation.

These differences in toe direction highlight several key aspects of karate's development. They reflect distinct lineage traditions (e.g., Kiba Dachi often linked to Shuri-te and Shiko Dachi to Tomari-te influences), emphasize various martial applications (such as rotational power, stability, or mobility), and illustrate the historical evolution of karate as masters adapted forms to their preferences and pedagogical needs. Ultimately, while personal preference and biomechanics can influence the choice of stance, ensuring proper knee alignment is essential for injury prevention.

At its core, Naihanchi dachi, regardless of toe variation, focuses on hip engagement, grounded power, and lateral mobility. The kata's movements emphasize rooted shifting, generating torque through the hips, and coordinating upper and lower body movements. Common sequences include inward blocks, backfists, cross-palm strikes, elbow strikes, and palm-up limb manipulations. Its application (bunkai) ranges from grappling counters to joint locks and takedowns, often targeting vulnerable areas. The lateral stepping inherent in the kata is crucial for maintaining centerline dominance and adjusting effectively in confined spaces. Additionally, muchimi, breath control, and cycles of tension and relaxation are incorporated into Naihanchi training, fostering full-body awareness and explosive stability through a strong focus on spinal alignment and leg tension.

Naihanchi's Diverse Paths

Naihanchi's fundamental importance is underscored by its numerous variations across different karate styles, such as Shotokan (called Tekki), Shoryun, Motobu-ryu, and Matsubayashi-ryu. While many Shuri-based schools preserve its segmented three-form structure, some systems influenced by Naha-te traditions maintain a singular, unified version of the kata. Itosu Anko's pedagogical influence notably led to the simplification and segmentation of Naihanchi, making it more accessible for public school instruction. In contrast, Motobu Choki emphasized the kata's direct combative applications, arguing that mastery of Naihanchi alone could be sufficient for real fighting, stressing that kata serves as a living record of combative principles rather than merely a performance art. He primarily transmitted this philosophy through oral teaching, resulting in subtle differences in execution compared to other lineages. Another influential master, Nagamine Shoshin, regarded Naihanchi as foundational for all karate movement, encouraging students to revisit its apparent simplicity for a deeper understanding.

Beyond individual interpretations, Naihanchi's core biomechanical principles—especially its lateral movements and powerful structure—significantly influenced later kata designs, most notably the Pinan series. These principles continue to inform close-range applications even in systems like Goju-ryu. Unfortunately, in modern sport karate, the crucial emphasis on bunkai for kata like Naihanchi is often overshadowed, with the focus shifting primarily toward precise form execution rather than the kata's deeper combative essence.

Naihanchi's Lasting Impact

The Naihanchi stand as some of Okinawa's most enduring kata; a seeming paradox of simplicity and complexity. Though its origins remain debated, its value is universally acknowledged as both a primer and a master form. Naihanchi demands, and rewards, decades of study as within its rooted stance and lateral stride lie the secrets of stability, sensitivity, and martial truth passed down through generations.

PINAN SERIES
OKINAWA'S PEACEFUL FORMS

Introduction to Pinan

In the global landscape of Karate, few kata are as widespread, foundational, and significant as the Pinan (平安) series. For countless practitioners around the world, these five forms represent their first introduction to the structured movements of Karate. They may appear simple, but they conceal a profound purpose; the Pinan kata are not merely beginner exercises, but they serve as a critical transition point in the history of Okinawan martial arts, marking the shift from a secretive, privately transmitted combat art to a systematized discipline taught to the public.

This exploration will examine the origins of the Pinan kata, the visionary master who created them, their unique technical contributions, and their lasting legacy as the foundation of modern Karate education.

Exploring the Essence of Pinan

- **Traditional Notation:** 平安 (Pinan; in mainland Japanese reading: Heian).
- **Script Breakdown:**
  - 平 "flat/even";
  - 安 "peace."
  - Together: "peaceful mind/peace and safety."
- **Core Meaning:** "Tranquil/peaceful mind."
- **Modern Interpretations:** Framed pedagogically as "peaceful" forms to instill calm foundations.
- **Conflicting Ideas & Origins:** Not contested; Itosu named the series c. 1900s; Funakoshi used the On-yomi (Heian).

The name "Pinan" (平安) carries a dual meaning that reflects the transformative era of its creation. It is made up of two Japanese characters: "Hei" (平), which means "peace" or "level," and "An" (安), meaning "safety" or "calm." Together, "Heian" (as it is known in mainland Japan) or "Pinan" (in Okinawan pronunciation) translates to "Peaceful Mind" or "Safety and Peace."

This dual interpretation is crucial for understanding the purpose of the kata. On one side, it emphasizes the importance of developing a calm and peaceful mindset through the disciplined practice of Karate, which fosters inner tranquility and self-control; key philosophical tenets of the art. On the other side, it subtly hints at achieving "safety and peace" as a practical outcome of self-defense, suggesting that mastering these forms enables one to navigate the world safely.

This linguistic duality reflects a deliberate shift in the public perception of Karate during the early 20th century. As the art transitioned from being a clandestine means of self-defense to a recognized form of physical education, its focus expanded to include character development and societal harmony. Therefore, the name embodies both an educational purpose and a cultural aspiration, reflecting a time when Karate was being reframed for a modern, public audience.

Pinan's Historical Origins

In the twilight of the 19th century, as Okinawa stood at the crossroads of tradition and modernity, a visionary martial artist named Itosu Anko reshaped the soul of Karate with his creation of the Pinan Kata. Born in 1831, Itosu was no ordinary master. A scholar-official in the fading Ryukyu Kingdom and a direct disciple of the legendary Matsumura Sokon, he embodied a rare blend of intellectual rigor and martial prowess. His life unfolded during a transformative era, as the Meiji Restoration swept through Japan, annexing Okinawa and ushering in sweeping societal changes. It was in this crucible of change that Itosu forged the Pinan kata, a series of forms that would become a cornerstone of modern Karate.

Itosu's vision was revolutionary yet pragmatic; he transformed Karate from an exclusive art for warriors into a universal discipline that could strengthen both body and character. With Okinawa's integration into Japan, the old ways of secretive, combative training were at odds with the new push for standardized education and military readiness. Recognizing that Karate's survival depended on its accessibility, Itosu set out to create a set of kata that could be taught to the masses, particularly to children in Okinawa's burgeoning public school system. Between 1902 and 1907, as Karate was officially introduced into schools, the Pinan kata were born; five forms designed to be safe, approachable, and pedagogically sound.

These kata were a deliberate departure from the complex and often dangerous forms of the past, such as Kusanku and Passai, which Itosu had mastered under Matsumura's tutelage. Drawing inspiration from an enigmatic form known as "Channan," a kata shrouded in mystery, with no surviving definitive version, Itosu wove together elements of these older traditions. He distilled their essence, simplifying intricate sequences into linear, manageable movements that emphasized fundamental body mechanics. This wasn't mere reduction, but a masterful synthesis, preserving the spirit of Okinawan Te while making it suitable for large-scale instruction. The result was a series of kata that instilled discipline, promoted physical health, and aligned with the educational ideals of the time, transforming Karate from a clandestine art of self-defense into a vital part of civic life.

Itosu's innovation wasn't just technical, it was cultural. By making Karate accessible, he ensured its survival in a world that might have otherwise left it behind. His Pinan kata became a bridge, guiding beginners toward the deeper, more intricate forms of the art while embedding Karate into the fabric of Okinawan society, and the legacy of the Pinan kata extended beyond Itosu's era, finding a home in the teachings of later masters.

Soken Hohan (1889–1982), a steadfast guardian of the Matsumura Seito lineage, and his student Kise Fusei (born 1935) embraced the Pinan series, integrating it into their system. They recognized its value as a structured pathway, guiding students from basic techniques to the advanced, traditional kata of their lineage. Even in a style rooted in the old ways, the Pinan kata proved indispensable, a testament to Itosu's enduring genius.

Through the Pinan kata, Itosu Anko didn't just preserve Karate, he redefined it. His work ensured that an ancient martial tradition could thrive in a modern world, its movements echoing through dojos across generations, a living legacy of a master who saw beyond his time.

Exploring Pinan's Wisdom

In the Pinan kata, practitioners are introduced to a foundational vocabulary of key techniques and their applications. Among these techniques, students learn a variety of basic blocks that not only teach fundamental defensive postures but also impart vital parrying actions alongside fundamental strikes. The focus here is on honing proper form, targeting accurately, and delivering impactful strikes.

Furthermore, the kata emphasizes smooth transitions between stances and techniques, allowing practitioners to learn to move efficiently. This flow is crucial for maintaining balance while shifting from defensive to offensive maneuvers. Although the bunkai introduced to beginners is often simplified, such as the sequence of a block followed by a punch, traditional interpretations reveal deeper layers of meaning, and many movements, when viewed through a combative lens, can be interpreted as joint locks, throws, or control techniques, illustrating the holistic nature of traditional Te.

While the internal aspects of Pinan, such as breath control and the concept of kime may not be emphasized as overtly as in other kata, they are subtly introduced; practitioners learn to synchronize their breath with movements, exhaling during exertion and inhaling in preparation, fostering not only rhythm and power but also cultivating the instantaneous tensing of the body at the moment of impact. Although Pinan does not delve into the deeper concepts of muchimi (sticky, viscous power) or kakei (continuous connection), it effectively lays the groundwork for these advanced principles through the development of fundamental body awareness and coordinated movement.

Pinan's Diverse Paths

The Pinan kata series, created by Itosu Anko, revolutionized Karate instruction by providing an effective teaching tool that spread widely across Okinawan schools, profoundly influencing the development of Karate in mainland Japan and beyond. This widespread adoption was driven by Itosu's introduction of the forms into Okinawan public schools, leading to various stylistic interpretations. Each interpretation reflects the unique teaching style, emphasis, and philosophical perspectives of different lineages.

As Karate expanded to mainland Japan, largely through the efforts of Itosu's students, such as Gichin Funakoshi, the Pinan kata became the foundational series for the emerging Japanese Karate styles. Although the core sequence of movements remains largely consistent, the execution, stances, and emphasis of these kata exhibit significant stylistic variations across various Okinawan and Japanese martial arts. These variations arose from several factors, with educational simplification being a primary driver, as masters adapted the forms to suit different teaching environments. The emphasis on specific principles and individual interpretations by masters, along with their unique physical attributes and understanding of the kata's combative intent, also played significant roles in shaping the versions transmitted through their lineages.

Funakoshi notably renamed the kata "Heian" (平安), using the Japanese pronunciation to integrate Karate into the Japanese Budo framework further while de-emphasizing its Chinese origins. The Shotokan version of the Heian kata, developed by Gichin Funakoshi, is characterized by strong, deep stances and powerful, linear movements, focusing on dynamic tension and crisp kime for decisive strikes and blocks.

In contrast, various Okinawan Shorin-ryu lineages, such as Matsubayashi-ryu and Shobayashi-ryu, embrace a different approach to the Pinan kata. Here, the emphasis is on more natural stances and fluid transitions, highlighting lighter and quicker movements that reflect Shorin-ryu's preference for agility and rapid changes in direction.

In the Matsumura Seito system, masters like Soken Hohan and Kise Fusei specifically adapted and integrated Pinan forms 3, 4, and 5 into their curriculum to accompany the versions of 1 and 2 passed down by Matsumura Nabe. They intended to create a structured and progressive learning path, guiding students from basic movements to more complex and combatively rich traditional kata of their lineage, such as Passai and Chinto. For them, these Pinan forms were essential preparatory exercises, instilling fundamental principles before progressing to the deeper applications found in older forms.

Regardless of their various interpretations, the Pinan kata series has profoundly impacted other forms and the overall martial arts curriculum. They have become the standard introductory series for countless Karate styles, influencing how subsequent kata are taught and understood. Their emphasis on standardized movements and clear educational progression laid the groundwork for the systematic teaching of Karate that is prevalent today.

Pinan's Lasting Impact

The Pinan kata represent a significant milestone in the history of Okinawan Karate, marking a crucial moment where tradition and modernization intersect. Created by Itosu Anko, these kata signal a deliberate shift from a secretive combat art to a structured and accessible discipline suitable for public education. Rather than being simplistic or basic, the five Pinan kata are meticulously designed gateways into deeply complex martial systems, showcasing a sophisticated approach to teaching.

FUKYUGATA

OKINAWA'S UNIFYING BASICS

Introduction to Fukyugata

In the vast and intricate annals of Okinawan Karate, few kata are as universally practiced, yet as profoundly misunderstood, as the Fukyugata series. Often casually dismissed as mere "beginner forms," these kata hold a unique and pivotal place in the modern history of Karate. They represent the very first concerted attempts to unify divergent styles under a shared pedagogical framework, a silent testament to a turbulent era of transition. Contrary to the common misconception that they are stripped-down, simplified remnants of more complex kata, the Fukyugata were, in fact, meticulously constructed. They were engineered to embody core principles of the art while simultaneously remaining accessible to novices, a delicate balance of simplicity and profound depth. This exploration delves into the multi-layered genesis of these forms, dissecting their technical DNA, and illuminating the influential figures who stood behind their development, revealing a story far richer than surface appearances suggest.

Exploring the Essence of the Fukyugata

- **Traditional Notation:** 普及形 (also 普及型) "popularization form."
- **Script Breakdown:**
    - 普 "universal";
    - 及 "reach/spread";
    - 形/型 "form/kata."
- **Core Meaning:** "Standardized popularization kata."
- **Modern Interpretations:** Often linked to 1940s Okinawa school curricula (Nagamine's No. 1; Miyagi's No. 2).
- **Conflicting Ideas & Origins:** Names are consistent; later Miyagi's No. 2 was re-titled Gekisai in Goju circles (see below).

The very term "Fukyugata" (普及形) carries a weight of intent. It combines "Fukyu" (普及), meaning "to disseminate" or "to make universal," with "Gata" (形), the familiar word for "form" or "pattern." Together, Fukyugata denotes a "promotional" or "unifying" form, its nomenclature emphasizing function over strict lineage. These forms were not primarily aimed at preserving ancient, esoteric combative secrets, but rather at standardizing Karate instruction across the numerous burgeoning schools. The name itself, therefore, reflects both a clear intent to provide a common entry point for learning and a broader cultural and political mission to unify the island's divergent martial traditions during a period of escalating nationalistic pressures.

Fukyugata's Historical Origins

The genesis of the Fukyugata series is rooted in a specific historical moment, shaped by the vision and, at times, the reluctance of influential masters, and driven by the political currents of the time.

The "Who" behind these foundational forms are two of the most prominent Okinawan Karate masters of the early 20th century: Nagamine Shoshin and Chojun Miyagi. Nagamine, the esteemed founder of Matsubayashi-ryu, brought a strong emphasis on natural stances, brisk and efficient movements, and practical self-defense techniques to his creation, Fukyugata Ichi. His approach reflected the dynamic, external aspects often associated with Shorin-ryu. Miyagi, the revered founder of Goju-ryu, was responsible for Fukyugata Ni. His contribution subtly emphasized internal strength, the nuanced interplay of tension and relaxation, and structured breathing; foreshadowing the deeper internal work of his style's quintessential kata, Sanchin. The collaboration of these two giants, representing distinct stylistic lineages, underscores the project's unifying purpose.

Created in 1940, these forms were specifically commissioned by Gen Hayakawa, who served as the governor of Okinawa Prefecture at the time. This period was marked by escalating Japanese militarism and an increasing governmental concern over physical education and cultural unity across the Japanese prefectures, including the recently annexed Ryukyu Islands. Karate, which had once been cloaked in secrecy, was rapidly transitioning into the public sphere, particularly within the school system. For this widespread public instruction, uniform training tools were deemed essential, providing a standardized curriculum where none had existed before.

The Fukyugata thus served dual, yet interconnected, purposes. On one hand, they were designed as accessible, entry-level kata for young or inexperienced students, providing a gentle introduction to the physical demands and basic movements of Karate. On the other, and perhaps more profoundly, they functioned as symbolic bridges between otherwise distinct martial traditions. The official commissioning of these forms by the prefectural government signaled a significant shift in Karate's role in Okinawan society: it was moving beyond its primary function as a self-defense art and being integrated into the civic curriculum as a tool for physical and moral education for the masses.

While not derived wholesale from a single, pre-existing kata, the Fukyugata skillfully drew inspiration from a range of foundational forms, distilling their essence into accessible movements. Miyagi's Fukyugata Ni, for instance, later evolved into the Gekisai Dai Ichi and Ni kata within Goju-ryu, incorporating and expanding upon the principles of dynamic tension and structured breathing central to his style. Nagamine's Fukyugata Ichi, in turn, reflected simplified elements found in the Pinan and Naihanchi kata, structured specifically for clarity and uniformity, ensuring that beginners could grasp fundamental body mechanics without being overwhelmed by complexity.

Exploring Fukyugata's Wisdom

Despite their foundational status, the Fukyugata forms are far from simplistic in their underlying principles. They are meticulously designed to train core martial concepts, serving as a comprehensive primer for the aspiring practitioner.

At their heart, the Fukyugata forms emphasize natural stances, enabling beginners to develop crucial balance and coordination without forcing unnatural postures. The movements themselves are typically large and linear, promoting efficient motor learning and establishing fundamental power mechanics. This deliberate design ensures that students build a solid physical foundation before progressing to more intricate or subtle techniques.

While seemingly basic, these forms subtly embed essential blocks, strikes, and transitions. Their bunkai (application) often includes straightforward counters to grabs and punches, designed to teach fundamental timing, targeting, and the concept of blocking and immediately countering. However, for the discerning practitioner and in certain traditional schools, these techniques hold deeper layers of meaning. They can also be interpreted to reveal applications involving joint locks or throws, skillfully obscured within what appear to be simple linear strikes and pivots. This layered interpretation speaks to the profound depth embedded even in these "beginner" forms.

The internal aspects, though perhaps less overtly emphasized for novices, are subtly present within the Fukyugata. Miyagi's version, Fukyugata Ni, for example, quietly includes elements of breath control and dynamic tension, serving as a gentle prelude to the deeper internal work found in the Goju-ryu kata such as Sanchin. Nagamine's Fukyugata Ichi, conversely, emphasizes a distinct rhythm and crisp kime (focus), aligning with Shorin-ryu's preference for light, fast movement and muchimi (sticky, flowing power), where the body moves as a cohesive unit. These subtle inclusions ensure that even at a foundational level, students are exposed to the distinct internal flavors of their respective styles.

Fukyugata's Diverse Paths

The Fukyugata Ichi and Ni forms, once commissioned, were adopted widely across various Okinawan schools and subsequently found their way into mainland Japan, becoming a ubiquitous part of Karate training. Yet, their journey was not one of static replication; they evolved, influenced by the unique philosophies and pedagogical approaches of different lineages.

Miyagi Chojun, for instance, later revised his Fukyugata Ni, transforming it into the Gekisai Dai Ichi and Gekisai Dai Ni kata for his Goju-ryu system. These revisions deepened the forms, incorporating more explicit Goju principles of hard and soft, open and closed, and further refining the breath control and dynamic tension that were Miyagi's hallmarks. In the Kenshinkan system, a lineage rooted in Matsumura Seito, Kise Isao Sensei introduced his own variations, Fukyugata Ni and San. These adaptations of the original Fukyugata Ichi align with the core principles of Matsumura Seito, ensuring that even the most basic movements convey clear combative intent across various levels.

These major stylistic variations arose due to differing teaching philosophies, the desired outcomes of training (whether for sport, discipline, or practical combat), and evolving interpretations of Karate's overarching purpose. While some schools might prioritize the athletic or competitive aspects, others, like Kise Isao's Kenshinkan, viewed these foundational forms as a crucial means to instill core combative concepts early in a student's training. This adaptability and reinterpretation highlight the dynamic nature of tradition itself, where forms are not merely preserved but continually re-examined and refined to serve the evolving needs of the art and its practitioners.

The creation of the Fukyugata was not without its philosophical tensions, and anecdotes from the masters themselves provide a glimpse into these debates. It is said that Chojun Miyagi, a man deeply committed to the profound, internal aspects of Goju-ryu, somewhat reluctantly developed his version of Fukyugata Ni. He reportedly expressed concern that such oversimplification, designed for mass instruction, would inevitably obscure the deeper essence of true Karate, fearing a dilution of the art's profound combative and philosophical core. Nagamine Shoshin, by contrast, embraced the challenge with a different perspective. He saw Fukyugata Ichi not as a diluted form, but as a crucial bridge to deeper learning, a necessary step to bring the art to a broader audience while still laying a solid foundation for future mastery. These differing approaches underscore the careful thought and, at times, internal struggle that accompanied the modernization of Okinawan Karate.

The Fukyugata's Lasting Impact

The Fukyugata forms stand at a pivotal crossroads of tradition and modernization in Okinawan Karate. Their creation marked a significant moment when the art, once shrouded in secrecy, sought structure, public visibility, and broader accessibility. Far from being shallow or merely rudimentary, these kata serve as carefully constructed gateways into profoundly complex martial systems. They embody the philosophical tensions inherent in any living tradition: the delicate balance between simplification for dissemination and the rigorous preservation of core principles, between individual stylistic expression and the unifying drive for a shared martial identity.

Today, the Fukyugata remain indispensable to Karate education worldwide, valued not only for their technical instruction but also for the rich historical narrative they represent. They are a testament to a martial tradition that, with foresight and adaptability, stepped forward to meet the needs of a changing world. In their elegant simplicity, they continue to guide countless practitioners, embodying the enduring spirit of Okinawan Karate and its timeless journey.

GEKISAI

OKINAWA'S STRIKING POWER

Introduction to Gekisai

Often underestimated due to its status as a beginner kata, Gekisai Dai Ichi holds an important place in the evolution of modern Okinawan Karate. Created as Fukyugata Ni by Chojun Miyagi in the early 1940s, it was part of a broader educational reform aimed at simplifying Goju-ryu training for school-aged youth while preserving its core principles. This kata, frequently misunderstood as merely a stepping stone to more advanced forms, actually embodies essential components of Miyagi's hard-soft philosophy and strategic body mechanics.

In this discussion, we will examine the creation, structure, and significance of Gekisai Dai Ichi. We will explore how it balances accessibility with depth, analyze key technical elements and variations, and place it in a historical context as a tool for national identity, physical education, and the preservation of martial arts.

Exploring the Essence of Gekisai

- **Traditional Notation:** 撃砕 (Gekisai); as kata: 撃砕第一/第二.
- **Script Breakdown:**
  - 撃 "strike/attack";
  - 砕 "smash/crush."
- **Core Meaning:** "Attack and smash/destroy."
- **Modern Interpretations:** Read as "pulverize" in some dojo vocab; created for robust basics.
- **Conflicting Ideas & Origins:** Title is stable; context sometimes discussed vis-à-vis 1940s public-school/standardization aims.

Between its creation in 1940 and the addition of the form to the regular curriculum of his dojo in 1948, Miyagi renamed the kata Gekisai Dai Ichi. The term "Gekisai" (撃縋) is often translated as "attack and destroy" or "demolish and smash," reflecting an aggressive intention behind its design.

The characters can also be interpreted more subtly: "Geki" (撃) means to strike or attack, while "Sai" (縋) conveys the idea of breaking through or subduing. This name indicates Miyagi's intention to create a form that emphasizes decisiveness and assertiveness—qualities that are ideal for fostering a martial spirit in youth.

Unlike many traditional Okinawan kata, which are named after specific places or have influences from China, Gekisai follows a straightforward Japanese naming convention. This suggests a shift toward national standardization and a broader educational appeal during the early Showa era, highlighting its role as an introductory yet serious training form.

Gekisai's Historical Origins

In the early 20th century, Chojun Miyagi (1888–1953), the visionary founder of Goju-ryu, developed a martial art that combined the internal practices of Chinese martial traditions with the practical combat techniques of Okinawan Naha-te. Influenced by his training with masters like Ro Ro Ko in China, Miyagi created a system that harmonized hard and soft principles; evident in technique, breath, and mindset. This dynamic balance became the hallmark of Goju-ryu.

In 1940, as Karate was transforming to align with Japan's nationalistic and educational agendas, the Karate-do Spececial Comittee was formed to incorporate Karate into school curricula, commissioning simplified kata to teach martial fundamentals to a broader audience. This led to the creation of the Fukyugata forms, one of which Miyagi would rename Gekisai Dai Ichi.

Miyagi designed Gekisai Dai Ichi as an approachable introduction for untrained youth, serving as a gateway to the more complex traditional kata like Sanchin and Seisan. The form emphasized linear motion, strong stances, and straightforward striking combinations, making it an ideal tool for instilling martial discipline while preserving Goju-ryu's internal principles. Despite its simplicity, Gekisai Dai Ichi retained the rooted stances and controlled breathing characteristic of Sanchin, reflecting Miyagi's commitment to depth even in introductory forms.

Its structure also exhibited subtle influences from the Pinan forms of Shorin-ryu, likely acknowledging shared goals of pedagogical simplification across Karate styles. Through clear transitions between sanchin-dachi (hourglass stance) and zenkutsu-dachi (forward stance), Gekisai Dai Ichi showcased Miyagi's brilliance in synthesizing traditional martial rigor with the practical needs of modern training, ensuring that even beginners could connect with the profound legacy of Goju-ryu.

Applying Gekisai's Combat Wisdom

The kata emphasizes zenkutsu-dachi (front stance) and sanchin-dachi (hourglass stance), training both external structure and internal alignment. The stance shifts train adaptability and grounded movement, Teaching forward momentum, rooted stability, and explosive linear techniques. With signature sequences that begin with a down-block, known as gedan-barai, which is typically followed by a powerful reverse punch, or gyaku-zuki. Another effective combination features a front kick, or mae-geri, that leads into a backfist strike, called uraken. Additionally, an elbow strike, referred to as empi, can be seamlessly integrated with transitional movement for greater versatility in combat situations.

Each of these techniques can be understood and applied in different contexts within a fight. For instance, the down-block may serve as a limb-clearing motion, allowing the practitioner to create space or disrupt an opponent's attack. The follow-up backfist can act as a response to destabilize an opponent further after they've lost their balance. Similarly, the elbow strike can be utilized as an effective weapon in close-range scenarios or to facilitate entry into a grappling clinch.

Despite the apparent simplicity of these kata, they hold deep layers of meaning and application. This is particularly true when analyzed through the lens of Goju-ryu, which emphasizes the effectiveness of techniques used at close distances. Many interpretations, or bunkai, arise from this approach, highlighting the depth and adaptability of traditional martial arts.

While less intense than Sanchin in breath discipline, it introduces foundational timing between exhale and exertion, laying the groundwork for deeper internal practice by introducing basic kime (focus), chinkuchi (explosive power), and breath control.

Gekisai's Diverse Paths

Though Gekisai Dai Ichi is a foundational kata in Goju-ryu that serves as a cornerstone for martial arts training, its influence extends beyond its origins, impacting systems like Kenshinkan and Kyokushin Karate, where it appears with slight variations in tempo and stance. Some schools modify its movements, adjusting for speed or tailoring them for tournament effectiveness, reflecting their unique priorities.

Traditional dojos emphasize internal alignment and controlled breathing, grounding the kata in disciplined precision. In contrast, sport-oriented schools focus on explosiveness and visually striking forms, prioritizing dynamic performance. Even transitions between stances, such as from sanchin-dachi to zenkutsu-dachi, vary across dojos, shaped by lineage traditions and biomechanical preferences.

As a precursor to more advanced forms, Gekisai Dai Ichi lays the groundwork for Gekisai Dai Ni, which builds on its simplicity by incorporating turning transitions and open-hand techniques. Its accessible structure makes it an essential stepping stone, preparing practitioners for the complexities of katas like Saifa and Seiyunchin. This solidifies its role as a vital entry point into the deeper layers of Goju-ryu training.

Gakisais Lasting Impact

Gekisai Dai Ichi is not merely an introductory kata but a precise and intentional distillation of Goju-ryu's core. Designed to teach structure, intention, and resilience, it serves as a rite of passage into a deeper understanding of Karate. By balancing simplicity with foundational depth, Miyagi's creation continues to shape generations of practitioners, proving that strength in Karate lies not in complexity, but in the refinement of principle.

TENSHO
OKINAWA'S FLOWING HANDS

Introduction to Tensho

In the vast and intricate world of Okinawan Karate, some kata are well-known for their powerful and dynamic movements, while others hold a more subtle yet equally significant meaning. Among these, Tensho stands out as a unique reflection of the deeper, internal aspects of the art. At first glance, it may seem deceptively simple. Still, it embodies a sophisticated blend of breath, tension, and fluid motion, showcasing a profound connection to the philosophical foundations of Okinawan martial traditions. This exploration examines the origins of Tensho, the visionary masters who contributed to its development, and its lasting legacy as a fundamental practice for internal cultivation.

Exploring the Essence of Tensho

- **Traditional Notation:** 転掌 (Tenshō).
- **Script Breakdown:**
  - 転 "turn/rotate";
  - 掌 "palm."
- **Core Meaning:** "Rotating/Turning Palms."
- **Modern Interpretations:** Often linked to Bubishi/Rokkishu hand methods; "soft" complement to Sanchin.
- **Conflicting Ideas & Origins:** Attributions to Miyagi, name, and etymology are standard.

The name Tensho itself suggests its essence: "revolving" or "changing" hands, indicating a continuous, fluid motion that is both defensive and offensive, adaptable yet steadfast. This kata emphasizes circularity, smooth transitions from soft to hard, and the cultivation of internal energy (ki); qualities that set it apart from many of Karate's more linear forms. As a practitioner, one is particularly drawn to its introspective nature, perceiving in its movements a deep meditation on the balance of power and control.

Tensho's Historical Origins

The creation and popularization of Tensho are closely connected to the insights and dedication of several key figures in the history of Okinawan and Japanese martial arts. Their diverse backgrounds and shared commitment to the deeper principles of the art led to the development of this unique kata.

The primary developer of Tensho was Chojun Miyagi, the revered founder of Goju-ryu Karate. Miyagi Sensei, a profound scholar and practitioner, devoted a significant portion of his life to the in-depth study of Chinese martial arts, particularly those from Fujian Province, which

25

emphasized internal cultivation, dynamic tension, and refined breathing methods. Tensho was Miyagi's direct attempt to integrate these internal principles into a kata that would complement the hard, external conditioning of Sanchin. While Sanchin focuses on rootedness, linear power, and isometric tension, Tensho explores fluidity, circularity, and the dynamic interplay of tension and relaxation. Miyagi's genius lay in creating a form that, through precise movements and synchronized breathing, allowed practitioners to cultivate ki and develop a soft power adaptable to any situation. For him, Tensho was not just a sequence of movements but a moving meditation, a pathway to internal mastery.

Miyagi's close friend and esteemed collaborator, Kenwa Mabuni, the founder of Shito-ryu, also played a significant role in the development and dissemination of Tensho. Mabuni Sensei possessed an encyclopedic knowledge of kata, having studied under both Itosu Anko (Shorin-ryu) and Higashionna Kanryo (Naha-te, the precursor to Goju-ryu). His broad understanding of various martial traditions undoubtedly influenced the refinement of Tensho, ensuring its adaptability and technical richness. Mabuni's meticulous approach to kata preservation and his willingness to integrate diverse influences helped solidify Tensho's place within the broader Karate landscape, even beyond Goju-ryu.

Later, a figure from a different lineage, Masutatsu Oyama, the founder of Kyokushinkai Karate, held Tensho in exceptionally high regard. This may seem surprising given Kyokushinkai's reputation for brutal, full-contact sparring and emphasis on external power. However, for Oyama Sensei, Tensho was profoundly important precisely because it provided the necessary internal balance to meet the rigorous physical demands of his style. He understood that true power came not just from external force but from a deep internal wellspring. Tensho's dynamic breathing and focus on ki cultivation offered his practitioners a means to develop resilience, mental fortitude, and a deeper connection to their own bodies, preventing them from becoming merely "muscle-bound" fighters. For him, it was the yin to Kyokushinkai's yang, essential for complete martial development.

Exploring Tensho's Combat Wisdom

To truly understand Tensho, one must explore its intricate technical and philosophical foundations, examining its unique characteristics and its relationship with other fundamental forms. A significant area of research related to Tensho is its connection to the "Rokkishu" (六機手), which can be found in the Bubishi, a classical text on Okinawan martial arts. The "Rokkishu" outlines six principles of hand techniques, represented by the dragon, tiger, leopard, crane, snake, and bear. These principles emphasize the development of specific internal qualities and applications. The movements in Tensho, particularly its open-hand techniques and fluid transitions, are believed to embody these "Rokkishu" principles. This allows practitioners to cultivate various types of power and adapt to different combative scenarios, translating ancient wisdom into dynamic motion.

Additionally, Tensho is often regarded as a "companion kata" to Sanchin, especially within Goju-ryu. While Sanchin focuses on developing a strong, rooted stance, achieving linear power, and the ability to absorb and deliver impact with significant isometric tension, Tensho complements it by emphasizing dynamic breathing, fluid circular movements, and generating power through relaxation and precise body rotation. Together, these two kata represent the hard and soft elements, the yin and yang, of Goju-ryu's combative philosophy. Practicing both kata fosters a holistic development of martial attributes, teaching practitioners to be both immovable and adaptable, powerful and yielding.

The specifics of Tensho's dynamic breathing and open-hand techniques are central to its internal cultivation. The breathing in Tensho is often deep and controlled, synchronized with the movements to facilitate the cultivation and circulation of ki. Unlike the closed-fist strikes of many Karate forms, the open-hand techniques emphasize gripping, tearing, pressing, and manipulating an opponent's balance. These techniques have their roots in the rare "Paipuren" form, a Chinese White Crane kata that Miyagi Sensei studied and that heavily influenced Tensho's unique methodology. The "Paipuren" lineage emphasizes soft, flowing movements and close-quarters manipulation, principles that Miyagi masterfully integrated into Tensho, transforming it into a powerful self-defense tool that relies on finesse and internal power rather than brute force.

Tensho's Lasting Impact

Through its intricate design and profound philosophical depth, Tensho stands as a testament to the internal dimensions of Okinawan Karate. It is a kata that continues to challenge and enlighten practitioners, unveiling the hidden layers of strength and adaptability within the art.

KANSHIWA

OKINAWA'S CIRCULAR STRENGTH

Introduction to Kanshiwa

Kanshiwa is often overlooked and dismissed by some as merely a "beginner's kata" or an introductory form within the Uechi-ryu curriculum. However, such dismissal is a mistake. Beneath its seemingly simple exterior lies a structure rich in layered meaning, historical significance, and technical insight. In many ways, Kanshiwa serves as a gateway: transitioning from static posture to flowing combat, from foundational breathing to dynamic motion, and from homage to innovation.

Created in the mid-20th century by Uechi Kanei, the son of the legendary Uechi Kanbun, Kanshiwa was designed to provide students with their first real challenge after mastering the stationary power and posture of Sanchin. Additionally, it serves as a philosophical bridge—an act of remembrance that connects the Chinese roots of Okinawan karate with its modern evolution. This chapter explores the origins, structure, and enduring significance of Kanshiwa in Okinawan karate as both a technical tool and a tribute to the legacy that gave rise to Uechi-ryu.

Exploring the Essence of Kanshiwa

- **Traditional Notation:** Commonly written カンシワ; some lineages coin kanji like 完子和, but usage isn't standardized.
- **Script Breakdown:** (If kanji used) 完 "complete"; 子 "child"; 和 "harmony/peace"—but most treat it as a coined name combining "Kan-" (Kanbun) and "-shiwa" (Shushiwa/Zhou Zihe).
- **Core Meaning:** A commemorative/constructed title; not a classical word.
- **Modern Interpretations:** Memorializes Kanbun Uechi and (alleged) teacher Shushiwa.
- **Conflicting Ideas & Origins:** Kanji assignments differ across Uechi groups; katakana use acknowledges the neologism.

The name Kanshiwa (完子和) symbolizes a fusion that honors the founders of Uechi-ryu. The first kanji, 完 (Kan), pays tribute to Uechi Kanbun, the founder of the style. The remaining two characters, 子 (Shi) and 和 (Wa), are taken from the name of Kanbun's Chinese mentor, Shushiwa (周子和). This combination serves as an act of veneration, recognizing both the Okinawan founder and his Chinese teacher.

Earlier versions of the kata were called Kanshabu, based on an older romanization of Shushiwa's name as "Shushabu." However, in the early 1970s, a correction in Chinese transliteration led to the more accurate rendering, Kanshiwa. While most modern lineages now use this updated name, some still retain Kanshabu, especially in variant systems or traditionalist circles.

Linguistically, the name does not carry a direct martial meaning and is not descriptive like "Gekisai" or "Tensho." Instead, Kanshiwa serves as a marker of lineage, preserving the legacy of Uechi-ryu's creation story through daily practice.

Kanshiwa's Historical Origins

Kanshiwa was created in 1954 by Uechi Kanei, a forward-thinking martial artist who recognized the need for effective teaching tools in a rapidly modernizing Okinawa. While his father's martial art had been developed through rigorous training in Chinese settings and tested in military contexts, Kanei aimed to refine Uechi-ryu for a new generation of students, many of whom were non-combatants or school-aged.

Before Kanshiwa's introduction, beginners in Uechi-ryu transitioned directly from Sanchin, a tense, breath-focused form that emphasizes structure and stability, into more complex forms like Seisan. The difference in complexity between these forms was significant. Kanshiwa was designed to bridge that gap, providing students with a dynamic yet accessible kata that began to incorporate movement, distance, timing, and offense, all while reinforcing the principles of Sanchin.

Importantly, the kata was named to honor two foundational figures: Uechi Kanbun and Shushiwa. This naming not only paid tribute to their contributions but also emphasized Kanshiwa's role as a continuation of the shared martial exchange between Chinese and Okinawan traditions. In terms of teaching, Kanshiwa quickly gained widespread use; the Okinawan Prefectural Government even included it as one of the standard katas taught to school-aged children, ensuring its broad dissemination. Related styles, such as Koburyu, similarly adopted this form into their own curricula, further affirming its foundational significance.

Applying the Wisdom of Kanshiwa

Kanshiwa is a kata designed with pedagogical intent, aimed at bridging the gap between static foundational forms and dynamic advanced forms. It uses four core stances and introduces students to movement concepts that are not present in Sanchin, such as weight shifting, closing distance, evasion, and striking in sequence. While it is simplified compared to senior forms, Kanshiwa remains technically rich.

This kata introduces several blocking techniques, including the Open-Hand Circle Block, which teaches the principle of circular redirection. It also features the Partial Circle with Double Palm Strike, demonstrating how to layer defensive and offensive strategies, as well as a Pressing Block for intercepting low strikes. Kanshiwa includes Seiken Punches, which are distinctive in this context as they use standard fist punches rather than the more complex and potentially hazardous shōken (knuckle fist) strikes found in many Uechi-ryu forms. Additionally, the kata includes palm and elbow strikes for close-range engagement, along with two types of kicks to reinforce fundamental skills such as chambering, targeting, and balance recovery.

Students learn about kime, rhythm, and transitional timing, understanding not just what a technique is but also when and how it should be executed. The kata features two kiai points, strategically placed to emphasize and test energy management. Kanshiwa operates on three learning levels, each requiring progressively deeper control, fluidity, and internal connection. Despite its elementary design, its structured repetition provides an evolving roadmap for technical development.

While the bunkai of Kanshiwa is often presented in simplified forms for beginners, the kata itself is rich with realistic applications rooted in Okinawan self-defense principles. The initial blocks redirect force and create vital space for counterattacks. The Seiken punches serve either as direct counterattacks or suppressive strikes. The combinations of palm and elbow strikes are effective in close-range encounters and reflect typical responses in tuidi (grappling and joint manipulation). Moreover, the pressing blocks and kicks are strategically combined with off-line movement, suggesting a tactical approach to evading attacks followed by counterattacks that destabilize or clear the opponent. Advanced practitioners often revisit Kanshiwa to refine their timing and distancing, frequently uncovering subtle grappling layers in the transitional movements that link blocks and strikes.

Kanshiwa's Diverse Paths

Kanshiwa is widely recognized in mainline Uechi-ryu, but it appears in a modified form within systems like Koburyu, which have adapted it to meet their specific teaching goals. Since this kata has a relatively recent origin, it exhibits less stylistic variation compared to older forms such as Seisan or Kusanku.

Some branches of Uechi-ryu continue to use the older name, Kanshabu, which maintains a historical link to the original romanization of Shushiwa. These minor naming differences can reflect deeper ideological divisions between those who prefer to preserve traditional forms and those who seek updates for clarity or accuracy.

The change from shōken (knuckle fist) to seiken (standard fist) punches in Kanshiwa represents a deliberate pedagogical choice, highlighting a commitment to modifying traditional practices for the safety and understanding of beginners. This demonstrates the kata's adaptability and its role as an effective tool within a structured curriculum.

Kanshiwas Lasting Impact

Kanshiwa may be considered a "modern" kata by Okinawan standards, but it embodies its legacy with respect and humility. It serves as both a practical instructional tool and a symbolic gesture of honor, linking the founder of Uechi-ryu with the Chinese mentor who influenced him. Through its name and structure, it narrates a story of connection, progression, and responsibility.

Though its movements may appear simple at first glance, they contain the foundations of mastery. As a bridge kata, connecting static structure to dynamic motion, Sanchin to Seisan, and beginners to advanced practitioners, it has become an essential part of Uechi-ryu's internal philosophy.

Studying Kanshiwa allows one to gain deeper insights into lineage, movement, and the balance between preservation and innovation. Like all great bridges, it invites us to cross over and explore further.

SECTION II - INTERMEDIATE KATA

TRANSITIONS IN FORM, DEPTH IN FUNCTION

The kata grouped here as "intermediate" are neither modern performance pieces nor purely archaic rituals. They represent a shift from technical repetition to tactical integration. These forms introduce more complex transitions, directional changes, asymmetrical timing, and layered strategies. Practitioners are expected to begin thinking beyond the solo sequence, considering how these movements function under pressure, in motion, and within context.

Many of these forms, such as Seienchin, Sanseiryu, and Wanshu, were once regarded as advanced within their respective systems, often taught selectively and sometimes only after years of training. Their current classification as "intermediate" does not reflect a degradation of their value but rather a change in the scope of curricula and access to information. With more kata available to more students than ever before, intermediate forms now play a crucial role in bridging foundational drills with higher-order synthesis.

Another theme that emerges in this section is the internal complexity hidden by external simplicity. For instance, Chinto and Rohai may seem straightforward in rhythm or shape, but they contain embedded tactics such as controlling structure through angling, borrowing energy through deflection, and neutralizing posture through asymmetry.

While foundational kata teach you how to move, these kata explain why movement is necessary and how to respond when timing shifts, when the opponent does not cooperate, and when linear techniques alone are insufficient.

SEISAN

OKINAWA'S CLOSE-QUARTERS MIGHT

Introduction to Seisan

Seisan is one of the oldest and most widely practiced katas in Okinawan martial arts, yet it remains one of the most enigmatic. Found across several traditions, such Shuri-te, Naha-te, Tomari-te, and their modern descendants, this kata has been a cornerstone of martial training for generations. Often translated as "Thirteen," Seisan inspires theories that range from the mystical to the practical. Its movements are tightly structured, emphasizing close-range combat, dynamic transitions, and powerful strikes and locks. Despite its age, Seisan continues to evolve through the unique interpretations of each lineage.

This chapter will explore Seisan's complex origins, various stylistic expressions, and its deep technical and philosophical foundations. It will also highlight the often-overlooked contributions of women to Okinawan martial tradition, particularly focusing on Yonamine Chiru, whose association with the kata adds a compelling human element to its study.

Exploring Seisan's Essence

- **Traditional Notation:** 十三 (sometimes 十三手).
- **Script Breakdown:** 十三 "thirteen."
- **Core Meaning:** "Thirteen (hands/techniques)."
- **Modern Interpretations:** Number may denote tactics, counts, or symbolic numerology from Fujian boxing.
- **Conflicting Ideas & Origins:** Competing theories on what "13" encodes (techniques, steps, points); number-kata tradition is well attested.

As mentioned, the name "Seisan" is most commonly interpreted to mean "Thirteen," but its exact significance is a topic of debate. Some believe it refers to thirteen techniques, steps, or hands, while others think it has symbolic meaning in Chinese numerology, where the number thirteen can represent luck or completeness. Another theory links Seisan to the Chinese "Four Gate Hands," a form that may have been introduced to Okinawa by martial artists from Fujian.

The meaning of Seisan can vary depending on the school and historical context. Some styles maintain the numerical interpretation, while others explore phonetic or translational connections to Chinese forms. The ambiguity of the name reflects the kata's widespread adaptation and diffusion across different martial and cultural contexts.

Seisan's Historical Origins

Seisan is a cornerstone of Okinawan martial arts, likely emerging in the late 18th or early 19th century, before the formalization of modern karate styles. Its roots are deeply connected to the historical exchanges between Okinawa and Fuzhou, China, particularly within the traditions of the White Crane martial arts families. While there is no direct Chinese counterpart to Seisan, it is often associated with Southern Chinese "Four Gate" boxing. Its enduring survival and adaptation in Okinawa, despite the decline of its Chinese counterparts, highlight its significant cultural and combative relevance within Ryukyuan society.

Seisan was likely created or formalized as a comprehensive training tool designed to encapsulate essential close-range techniques, including strikes, throws, locks, and evasions, all within a single form. It served as a cohesive method for defense, internal conditioning, and the efficient transmission of core martial principles, acting as a vital bridge that connects foundational forms with more complex expressions of martial skill.

Key figures who played crucial roles in shaping the early development and philosophical undertones of Seisan inclue people like Takahara Peichin, Matsumuar Sokon, and his wife Yonamine Chiru. Takahara Peichin, an 18th-century Okinawan scholar and martial artist, was among the earliest individuals linked to Seisan and was the teacher of Sakugawa Kangi. His teachings emphasized a holistic union of ethics, martial practice, and cosmic philosophy, which profoundly influenced the depth found in kata like Seisan.

Another notable figure is Yonamine Chiru, the wife of Matsumura Sokon. Oral traditions suggest that Chiru actively trained in and contributed to the evolution of Seisan. A powerful, albeit folkloric, tale recounts her defending herself while carrying a child on her back, vividly reflecting the kata's practicality and effectiveness in close-quarters combat. Although a legend, this story beautifully symbolizes the resilience and tactical ingenuity often overlooked in martial history, embodying the spirit that Seisan sought to cultivate.

Applying Seisan's Combat Wisdom

A multifaceted cornerstone of Okinawan martial arts, the kata known as Seisan is renowned for its characteristic deep-rooted stances, its movements emphasizing short bursts of power, shifting angles, and sudden changes in energy, frequently incorporating lateral movements, body drops, and inward spirals.

Within its form, it encapsulates a comprehensive array of techniques designed for close-range combat; including close-range punches and palm strikes, low kicks and knee strikes, sweeps, takedowns, and hip throws, as well as joint locks and pressure point applications. At its heart, Seisan teaches principles of interception, disruption, and counteroffense with bunkai that often involves controlling the opponent's centerline, disrupting their posture, and executing decisive follow-up finishes; seamlessly integrating both striking and grappling within flowing transitions.

Beyond its physical applications, Seisan is crucial for developing internal mechanics. Breath control and kime are central, particularly in Naha-te and Uechi-Ryu versions of the kata, and practitioners cultivate robust rooting through the feet, which develop explosive stability. For many, Seisan marks their first genuine encounter with these deeper internal aspects of martial arts, moving beyond mere gross movement.

Seisan's Diverse Paths

The widespread adoption across different styles highlights Seisan's foundational importance, though it has seen various interpretations. Prominently preserved in Goju-Ryu, it emphasizes close-range techniques with strong tension and breath work. Shorin-Ryu and Isshin-Ryu feature more linear versions, blending Goju elements with Shuri-te precision. Uechi-Ryu presents a distinct structure, incorporating powerful knee strikes and a unique breathing rhythm. In Shotokan, Seisan was transformed into Hangetsu, characterized by its slower, tension-based movements. A lesser-known variant, Arakaki-no-Seisan, is considered by some to be closest to its original Chinese influences.

These variations underscore how each system adapted Seisan to reflect its unique technical emphases and stylistic teaching goals. Naha-te styles, for instance, focused on internal development, while Shuri-te traditions highlighted posture and speed, and Uechi-Ryu incorporated Sanchin-based rooting. Changes also stemmed from individual teachers' interpretations, specific teaching needs, or limitations in the transmission process over generations. Consequently, Seisan has served as a significant technical and philosophical link in many curricula, profoundly influencing later kata such as Seipai, Kururunfa, and Sanseiru, particularly within Goju-Ryu.

Seisan's Lasting Impact

Seisan serves as a martial arts bridge that connects various styles, generations, and cultural exchanges. Its lasting presence in Okinawan karate programs highlights its depth, adaptability, and realistic combat applications. Although its exact origins may be unclear, its effectiveness as a teaching tool and a test of skill is evident. Through Seisan, students not only learn physical techniques but also gain insight into the rich history of Ryukyuan martial culture.

PASSAI
OKINAWA'S EVASIVE MASTERY

Introduction to Passai

Mysterious, powerful, and deeply rooted in tradition, Passai, also known as Bassai in Japanese, stands as one of the most revered and widely practiced katas in Okinawan Karate. This kata is rich in history, layered with evolution, and steeped in combative strategy. Although often translated as "To Penetrate a Fortress," Passai represents much more than a mere display of strength; it serves as a study in utilizing structure, redirection, and subtle control to overcome overwhelming force.

This chapter will explore the origins and development of Passai, examine its technical diversity across different lineages, and unpack the philosophical strategies embedded in its execution. We will also investigate the kata's transformation through the teachings of masters such as Matsumura Sokon, Itosu Anko, and Funakoshi Gichin, analyzing how this form has evolved into both a repository of tradition and a practical tool for self-defense.

Exploring Passai's Essence

- **Traditional Notation:** 抜塞 or 披塞 (variant); modern Shotokan uses 披塞 (Bassai).
- **Script Breakdown:**
    - 抜/披 "to break through/penetrate, to uncloak";
    - 塞 "fortress/stronghold."
- **Core Meaning:** "Penetrate/Break through the fortress."
- **Modern Interpretations:** Imagery of breaching defenses; dai/shō versions differentiate teachings.
- **Conflicting Ideas & Origins:** Multiple historical spellings exist (Tomari/Shuri variants).

Considered one of the oldest forms in Okinawan karate, Passai holds a deep and complex history, with origins potentially traceable back to Chinese martial arts. This makes the tracing of its name problematic, as oral tradition significantly predates written records. While its roots are undoubtedly ancient, the earliest known written reference to Passai appears relatively recently, in a 1911 newspaper article in the Ryukyu Shimpo. This article reported that Kiyuna Taro Pēchin, a student of Matsumura Sokon, performed Passai during a Teacher School Karate Meeting. This, and other early mentions, including those in Gichin Funakoshi's 1922 book, used katakana (パッサイ).

Funakoshi later changed the name to Bassai (バッサイ) and assigned Kanji characters (抜塞) to it in 1935, a move intended to make the kata more culturally palatable for the Japanese mainland. The characters inherently convey a forceful strategy: 抜 (Batsu or Hatsu) means "to pull out" or "extract," while 塞 (Sai) refers to "fortress" or "obstruction." Together, they encapsulate the idea of overcoming adversity through decisive, explosive action and are commonly interpreted as "To Penetrate a Fortress" or "To Storm a Fortress." This powerful interpretation was popularized by Funakoshi himself, who adapted it as "Bassai."

However, another layer of speculation suggests that the name might phonetically derive from the Fujian dialect term for lion dance, pronounced "pa sai" or "phah sai." This connection offers an intriguing cultural dimension, hinting that Chinese performance traditions may have influenced specific movements or the overall spirit of this enduring form.

Passai's Historical Origins

Often theorized to contain influences from Chinese martial arts such as Leopard or Lion boxing, Wuxing Quan (Five Element Fist), or Fujian Crane, Passai was designed as a self-defense form rich in tactics for turning disadvantage into advantage. Its dynamic footwork, sharp angles, and explosive counters suggest it was intended to teach practitioners how to dismantle a stronger or more aggressive attacker using timing, structure, and strategy. While no direct Chinese version of Passai exists today, the kata retains strong echoes of Chinese tactical thinking.

While the exact origin of Passai is unclear, it is believed to have arrived in Okinawa during the 18th or early 19th century. Bushi Matsumura Sokon, a key figure in the development of Shuri-te, is often credited with introducing Passai to the island. Some traditions, however, suggest that Matsumura learned Passai from Oyadomari Peichin, a martial artist based in Tomari. Regardless of the specifics of its introduction, Matsumura's interpretation laid the groundwork for many subsequent variations and firmly established Passai within the Shuri-te lineage. Its evolution continued through the Meiji period and into modern times, as masters like Itosu Anko and Funakoshi Gichin included it in school curricula and training regimens.

Exploring Passai's Wisdom

Passai is a dynamic and comprehensive tactical system that goes far beyond mere striking to encompass a full spectrum of defensive applications. Practitioners of this kata fluidly transition between various stances, mastering swift angular redirection and developing powerful linear advances complemented by precise pivots, quick weight shifts, and strategic angled counters.

Central to Passai's tactical repertoire are techniques such as knife-hand blocks and strikes, which serve as versatile tools for both trapping opponents and causing limb damage. The kata's distinctive cross-stepping footwork is executed strategically for throwing techniques and evasive repositioning, highlighting the emphasis on dynamic movement, fluidity, and adaptability in combat. These techniques are particularly useful in close-range scenarios for entering an opponent's space, creating angles, executing throws and sweeps, twisting offline from strikes, and stomping or trapping an opponent's foot. This demonstrates a fusion of grappling and striking that is a hallmark of traditional Okinawan karate.

The kata also includes counter-grappling sequences that provide practical methods for escaping grips, employing techniques that involve dropping or pulling away, as well as shin blocks, leg hooks, and aggressive shuffles used to effectively disrupt an opponent's balance. Some interpretations of the kata explore weapon defense applications, particularly against the bo, which are examined through various interpretations, most notably within the context of Bassai Dai.

These diverse applications firmly establish Passai as more than just a striking form; it is a comprehensive self-defense "atlas" intended for deep study and understanding, rather than simple performance. Through rigorous practice, Passai cultivates essential internal qualities such as focused energy, rootedness, and fluid redirection. Its transitions from tension to sudden release effectively mirror a combative rhythm, demanding both explosive power and instantaneous control, thereby aligning with the principle of integrating hard and soft dynamics without rigid duality.

Passai's Diverse Paths

Passai has a rich history, featuring over thirty recorded variations that showcase the unique insights of its masters and the regional traditions from which they emerged. Among these variations, Matsumura no Passai is notable for its distinct "Chinese" influence, reflecting deep historical roots. In contrast, Oyadomari no Passai presents a softer, more flowing interpretation closely related to Tomari-te. Itosu no Passai is well-known for its educational framework, famously divided into Passai Dai and Passai Sho, emphasizing a structured progression of learning.

Other important variations include Chibana no Passai, Motobu no Passai, Kyan no Passai, and Tawada no Passai, each contributing unique technical elements and collectively enriching the diversity and depth of Passai as a martial art.

These variations are not arbitrary; they arise from a combination of instructional needs, individual master insights, and distinct stylistic interpretations. For example, Itosu created Passai Sho as a stepping stone to the more comprehensive Passai Dai. Later, Funakoshi adapted both for the Shotokan style, renaming them Bassai Dai and Bassai Sho, while modifying their rhythm and stances to make them more accessible to modern practitioners. The dynamic movements and sophisticated structural tactics of Passai have significantly influenced the development of other kata, inspiring numerous adaptations across systems such as Shito-Ryu, Shotokan, and Isshin-Ryu. Its lasting legacy is evident in these adaptations and the ongoing interpretations by practitioners worldwide.

Additionally, historical accounts and oral traditions suggest that Passai played a crucial role in Okinawan self-defense, with some traditions indicating that it was specifically designed to teach defense against armed attackers or even multiple assailants, while others state that it was practiced secretly during periods of weapon bans. Although concrete historical records from these early times are limited, the preserved complexity and practical depth of Passai strongly indicate its vital role in real-world defense scenarios.

Passai's Lasting Impact

Passai is more than just a kata; it represents a dynamic evolution of tactical practice. With its mysterious origins and transmission through the masters of Okinawa, Passai has spread globally, continuing to challenge and inspire martial artists. Rich in history and practical application, it serves as a powerful example of transforming adversity into triumph. For serious practitioners, Passai is a cornerstone of martial arts knowledge, embodying both the hidden strength and enduring spirit of Okinawa.

NIJUSHIHO / NISEISHI
OKINAWA'S 24 STEPS

Introduction to Nijushiho

Nijushiho ("Twenty-Four Steps") is an elegant and mysterious kata that stands out in both the Shotokan and Shito-ryu martial arts traditions. It is characterized by nuanced movements, spiraling energy, and strategic control. The kata features smooth transitions, coiling strikes, and a unique tempo that reward those who engage in deep study. While it is practiced less frequently than more foundational kata, Nijushiho provides a glimpse into older Chinese-Okinawan influences, emphasizing redirection, joint manipulation, and internal timing.

This chapter delves into the origins, techniques, and philosophical foundations of Nijushiho. We trace its development from the Okinawan kata Niseishi, credited to Arakaki Seisho, through the teachings of Funakoshi Gichin, Mabuni Kenwa, and Nakayama Masatoshi. This exploration highlights its refined evolution into a form that blends old-world complexity with the structure of modern karate.

Exploring Nijushiho's Essence

- **Traditional Notation:** 二十四歩 (Nijūshiho).
- **Script Breakdown:**
    - 二十四 "24";
    - 歩 "steps."
- **Core Meaning:** "24 steps."
- **Modern Interpretations:** Sometimes tied to Chinese numerology; "steps" may mean sequencing or tactical "paces."
- **Conflicting Ideas & Origins:** Stable title; explanations of "steps" vary by school.

The term "Twenty-Four Steps" directly translates from characters that break down to ni (二, meaning two), ju (十, meaning ten), shi (四, meaning four), and ho (歩, meaning steps). Although the kata's movement count does not always match exactly with the number 24, earlier Okinawan versions were referred to as Niseishi (二十四), which is a dialectical pronunciation of the same term.

The significance of the number 24 may refer to distinct techniques, directional changes, or symbolic principles, but there is no definitive interpretation. Some suggest that it relates to the number of potential targets or angles of attack, while others believe it holds numerological significance within Chinese cosmology.

Nijushiho's Historical Origins

The kata known as Niseishi, a direct precursor to modern Nijushiho, holds a significant and complex place in the history of karate. Its origins are often attributed to Arakaki Seisho (1840–1920), a prominent Okinawan martial artist believed to have introduced several influential kata to the island, including Unsu, Sochin, and Niseishi itself. These forms were likely inspired by various Chinese martial systems, with Dragon style and Fujian White Crane often cited as potential influences.

The Chinese connections are clearly evident in Nijushiho's flowing, spiraling hand motions, whipping strikes, and dynamic shifting stances. While exact correlations remain speculative, martial historians suggest that the kata may have deeper roots in older internal systems that prioritize breath, continuous flow, and integrated body structure rather than overt athleticism. The origins of this kata date back to the late 19th century, marking its emergence within the evolving landscape of Okinawan martial arts.

Exploring Nijushiho's Wisdom

Nijushiho appears to have been intended to serve as a sophisticated bridge between raw close-quarter fighting principles and refined internal motion. Its techniques are meticulously designed to emphasize limb control, trapping, and torque, making it ideal for self-defense in confined spaces or during grappling situations. The form rigorously encourages precision under pressure, prioritizes timing over raw speed, and fosters adaptability over rigid formality. This approach focuses on structural off-balancing and internal rhythm rather than relying on large, dramatic movements.

The kata features a comprehensive range of key techniques that demonstrate a deep understanding of combat applications. Practitioners utilize circular double-hand motions, which can serve as parries or joint manipulations, allowing for effective defensive strategies. Close-range confrontations are addressed with hiji ate, or elbow strikes, delivered from coiled positions for maximum impact. Additionally, the kata incorporates awase-zuki, a technique involving coordinated punches where one arm strikes while the other maintains control of the opponent. A distinctive technique, haishu uchi, or back-hand strikes, is also present, which is less commonly seen in many kata.

Moreover, the kata includes two yoko-kekomi, or side thrust kicks, believed to be later additions aimed at enhancing offensive capabilities. Within the flowing sequences, practitioners also discover wrist traps, arm drags, and chokes, suggesting that the kata was specifically designed with grappling-range defense in mind. Overall, these techniques reflect a well-rounded strategy that balances defensive maneuvers with effective offensive actions.

Nijushiho's Diverse Paths

The historical trajectory of this kata began with Arakaki and was passed on to students such as Higaonna Kanryo, who then transmitted it to Kenwa Mabuni. Mabuni played a crucial role in refining the form within his Shito-ryu style. From there, the kata reached Shotokan through

Funakoshi Gichin and his son, Funakoshi Yoshitaka (Gigo). Its formal integration into Shotokan's system occurred in the mid-20th century, during a period of widespread technical codification by the Japan Karate Association (JKA). In the postwar years, a significant moment of cross-style collaboration took place when Shotokan leaders like Nakayama Masatoshi and Obata Isao met with Kenzo Mabuni (Kenwa's son) to align their understanding of the kata, an effort instrumental in solidifying the standardized form known as Nijushiho today.

The kata's journey across various styles has resulted in distinct stylistic interpretations. Shito-ryu Niseishi retains a strong Chinese influence, characterized by an emphasis on fluidity and nuanced hand movements. In contrast, Shotokan's version, Nijushiho, is defined by a more linear approach, showcasing clearly defined movements and incorporating additional kicks along with a broader embusen. Wado-ryu Nijushiho uniquely merges the Shotokan framework with the softer transitions characteristic of Wado, creating a distinctive blend of styles. These variations primarily arise from the differing stylistic philosophies of the schools. For instance, Shotokan prioritizes long-range engagement and prominent form, naturally leading to more expansive and explicit movements, while Shito-ryu opts for a compact, circular approach that emphasizes fluidity. Some adaptations are also influenced by competition requirements or the need for clearer pedagogical techniques.

The complexity of Nijushiho has established it as a significant reference point in the borrowing of techniques for the creation of other kata. Its spiraling arm movements and strategies for close-range combat have left a lasting impact, shaping modern kata development and the interpretation of bunkai. Intriguing legends and anecdotes further enrich this kata's story, with some recalling Funakoshi Gigo's particular favor for Nijushiho due to its subtlety and control, viewing it as a bridge integrating older Okinawan traditions into contemporary Japanese karate. Others remember Nakayama's dedication to maintaining the kata's integrity while adapting it for a unified Shotokan practice, ensuring its relevance in the ever-evolving landscape of martial arts.

Nijushiho's Lasting Impact

Nijushiho is a kata of transition, bridging styles, ranges, and eras. Grounded in Okinawan tradition but influenced by modern practitioners, it preserves the intricate touch associated with older martial arts while also offering a refined exploration of timing, precision, and internal connection. For serious karateka, it presents a lasting challenge and serves as a quiet, spiraling path toward deeper understanding.

CHINTO

OKINAWA'S CRANE ART

Introduction to Chinto

Chinto, also known as Gankaku in Shotokan, is one of the more enigmatic and acrobatic kata in the Okinawan martial arts tradition. This kata is steeped in legend and is characterized by its unique technical movements, as well as its compelling history and tactical implications. Its most renowned technique is the striking one-legged stance, which creates a vivid visual impact. However, it is the kata's intricate strategic evasions, sharp angles, and deceptive rhythms that truly establish it as a distinctive pillar in classical training.

This chapter delves into Chinto's obscure historical roots, its various interpretations across different lineages, and the legend of the mysterious Chinese martial artist who may have inspired it. We will examine the kata's sophisticated body mechanics, evasive tactics, and legacy, drawing insights from the teachings of notable figures such as Matsumura Sokon, Anko Itosu, Chotoku Kyan, and others who have contributed to its diverse forms.

Exploring Chinto's Essence

- **Traditional Notation:** 鎮東 (Chintō); Shotokan rename: 岩鶴 (Gankaku, "crane on a rock").
- **Script Breakdown:**
    - 鎮 "to quell/calm";
    - 東 "east."
- **Core Meaning:** Often glossed "fighter/battle to the east," or "calming the east."
- **Modern Interpretations:** Associated with the "one-leg" crane imagery in Gankaku.
- **Conflicting Ideas & Origins:**
    - "Chintō/Annan" as a person vs. directional title;
    - Funakoshi's rename avoids explicit Chinese allusions.

The name Chinto (鎮東), often translated as "Fighter to the East," "Calming the East," or sometimes "Eastward Calmer," carries powerful connotations. The kanji used in the name conveys this dual interpretation: 鎮 (chin) means "to calm" or "to suppress," while 東 (to) simply means "east."

The earliest known references to the Chinto kata were written in katakana, (ナイハンチ). The first recorded mention appeared in a 1914 newspaper article by Gichin Funakoshi. This article, based on accounts from his teacher Anko Asato, discusses individuals who received instruction from a castaway from Anan in Fuzhou, China, suggesting a direct connection to Chinese martial arts. Funakoshi's article also references figures like Gusukuma and Kanagusku in relation to Chinto, and mentions Matsumora and Oyadomari in connection with another kata, Chinti. This indicates that, regardless of its initial spelling, the kata was already well-known within the foundational Tomari-te and Shuri-te schools of karate.

The original name, Chinto, underwent a significant transformation under Funakoshi Gichin. In his effort to adapt karate for a mainland Japanese audience, Funakoshi renamed the kata Gankaku (岩鶴), which means "Crane on a Rock." This change was motivated by both political and aesthetic reasons. Politically, the renaming served to distance the kata from its overt Chinese origins during a time of rising anti-Chinese sentiment in Japan. Aesthetically, the new name highlighted the distinctive crane-like posture that is a prominent feature in Shotokan's interpretation of the kata.

Whether viewed as a "calming force" facing east or as a symbolic "crane on a rock" embodying vigilance and balance, the kata's name, both in its Okinawan and Japanese forms, underscores Chinto's inherent dual nature: an art that is simultaneously graceful and dangerous, deeply rooted yet evasive, elusive yet ultimately decisive.

Chinto's Historical Origins

The kata known as Chinto holds a captivating origin story, traditionally attributed to a shipwrecked Chinese martial artist named Chinto or Annan, who supposedly landed off the Okinawan coast—perhaps near Tomari—in the late 18th or early 19th century. While this legend is difficult to definitively verify, its consistent presence across generations of oral traditions strongly suggests the kata's perceived foreign origin.

Chinto likely entered Okinawan martial practice during the early to mid-1800s, coinciding with the late Ryukyu Kingdom era. This period was characterized by heightened cultural and trade exchange with Chinese maritime visitors, particularly from Fujian province, and a growing concern over the role of martial arts under the ruling Satsuma clan. It was during this time that Sokon Matsumura, a pivotal figure in Shuri-te development, is frequently credited with learning Chinto—either directly from the legendary Chinese visitor or through intermediaries such as Gusukuma or Kanagusuku. Matsumura then ensured its transmission within the Shuri-te lineage. Later, Anko Itosu and Chotoku Kyan each received and further modified the kata, with Kyan's version becoming particularly associated with the Tomari lineage.

Chinto's unique design, characterized by its angular evasions, deceptive stances, and narrow embusen (floor pattern), strongly suggests it was developed for use in constrained or uneven environments, much like the rocky shorelines of Okinawa. It stands apart as not a "marching kata," but rather a sophisticated form focused on subtle redirection, unbalancing, and close-range control. This tactical philosophy bears a striking resemblance to southern Chinese styles such as Wu Zho Quan (Five Ancestors Fist), Crane Boxing, and Chuan Fa. While no direct Chinese prototype of Chinto exists today, its distinctive off-line tactics and circular entries carry the unmistakable signature of Fujianese martial thought.

Exploring Chinto's Wisdom

Chinto is a complex kata that skillfully combines advanced movement principles and characteristic stances aimed at improving a practitioner's balance and ability to evade attacks. One of its most significant positions, the Sagi Ashi Dachi, or Crane Stance, strongly emphasizes stability. The kata incorporates dynamic angular stepping and pivoting, allowing for quick changes in direction and enabling swift movements that facilitate rapid adjustments during combat, especially on uneven terrain.

The movements within the kata alternate between low and high levels, creating a vertical disruptiveness, while techniques prioritize deceptive footwork, meticulously designed to prompt an opponent's attacks or to create advantageous moments for off-angle counters. Practitioners effectively utilize one-legged pivots not only for evasion but also for skillfully redirecting an opponent's momentum. Moreover, techniques that involve grabbing and unbalancing the opponent further enhance control during confrontations.

Dynamic counters play a crucial role by allowing practitioners to evade attacks while striking simultaneously. These techniques are highly valued for teaching precise timing, enhancing structural integrity under pressure, and encouraging creative uses of balance and space. Internally, Chinto requires practitioners to develop precise kime, while also maintaining essential transitional control and core stability. This kata is instrumental in training explosive tension shifts while promoting a loose and responsive engagement. Ultimately, it cultivates technical power, refines internal rhythm, and hones intuitive timing.

At its core, Chinto is a deep exploration of maintaining balance under pressure. Its challenging one-legged pivots and quick changes in direction demand a unique combination of being grounded without being inflexible. Instead of promoting direct confrontation, Chinto emphasizes the importance of subtle avoidance, redirection, and strategic counterattacks. It embodies the principle of "soft overcoming the hard" in a dynamic and flowing manner. From both a literal and strategic perspective, Chinto prepares practitioners to adapt effortlessly to imbalance, whether it's the uneven physical terrain of a fight or the unpredictable actions of an opponent.

Chinto's Diverse Paths

The transmission history of Chinto reveals two main lineages, each with distinct characteristics. The Tomari version, often associated with the Matsumora lineage, emphasizes lateral movement and evasion. This style is typically practiced in various schools such as Matsubayashi-Ryu, Seibukan, and Shorinji-Ryu. In contrast, the Shuri version, linked to the Itosu lineage, tends to be more linear. This approach is expressed in styles like Shotokan, Shito-Ryu, and Wado-Ryu. Notably, Shotokan has adapted elements from this lineage, particularly through its kata Gankaku, which shifts the focus toward crane stance balance and visual elegance, embodying a refined aesthetic in its movements.

These variations reflect the unique pedagogical goals and stylistic values of each master. For example, Itosu likely simplified and structured the kata for broader school instruction, while Kyan, who trained under Kosaku Matsumora, preserved more of the kata's fluid and adaptive qualities. Chinto's dynamic influence extends beyond its direct lineages; it has impacted later kata that emphasize diagonal strategy and single-leg balance. Its technical DNA can also be observed in hybrid forms found in modern karate and Korean systems like Tang Soo Do, where it appears as Jin Do or Jin Tae.

Fascinating legends and anecdotes surround this kata, including stories that Chotoku Kyan particularly favored Chinto for its elusive strategies and nimble footwork. It is said that he trained his students on Okinawa's shoreline cliffs to simulate the kata's intended terrain, further highlighting its emphasis on adaptability in challenging environments.

Chinto's Lasting Impact

Chinto is a kata that exists in the space between legend and reality. It tells the story of a mysterious Chinese martial artist who was shipwrecked and has been interpreted and adapted by various Okinawan karate masters over time. Its distinctive movements, characterized by forward-leaning stances, sharp angles, and lateral evasions, set it apart from other katas. Additionally, its mythic origins and unique tempo make it one of the most recognizable forms in the classical kata repertoire.

The lasting significance of Chinto lies in its asymmetry, which can be observed in its strategic, geographical, and historical contexts. It can be seen either as a tribute to an enigmatic teacher or as a product of the rich cultural fusion found in coastal Tomari. Chinto invites ongoing reinterpretation: for some, it represents cross-cultural exchange, while for others, it serves as a study in strategic displacement and the disruption of balance. In any case, it is not only a combative form but also a reminder that much of Okinawa's martial heritage arrived not by design but through the tides of history.

KUSANKU

OKINAWA'S DYNAMIC REDIRECTION

Introduction to Kusanku

Few kata in the Okinawan tradition are as widely practiced yet as often misunderstood as Kusanku. This form is named after a visiting Chinese martial artist whose historical presence is mostly known through diplomatic notes and secondhand performances. Despite its unclear origins, Kusanku has become a foundational pillar of Okinawan karate and serves as a litmus test for transmission across nearly every major lineage.

Also known as Koshokun, this kata is among the longest and most complex forms in traditional Okinawan karate. It exists in various iterations across different styles, reflecting distinct lines of descent and teaching focuses. The kata combines low stances with evasive maneuvers and blends fluid transitions with explosive strikes. In Shotokan karate, it is referred to as Kanku ("Gazing at the Sky"), an aesthetic reinterpretation that hints at the kata's philosophical undertones.

Kusanku is not a singular form but rather a layered composite shaped by oral transmission, selective memory, and stylistic adaptations. By exploring its historical roots, symbolic elements, and technical expressions, we can understand how this kata evolved into both a technical blueprint and a cultural monument within karate.

Exploring Kusanku's Essence

- **Traditional Notation:** 公相君 (Kōshōkun/Kūsankū); Shotokan rename: 観空 (Kankū "viewing the sky").
- **Script Breakdown:**
  - 公相君 (title/name; Chinese envoy honorific);
  - 観 "view";
  - 空 "sky/void."
- **Core Meaning:** As Kankū: "Viewing the sky"; as Kūsankū: eponymous (linked to a figure).
- **Modern Interpretations:** Opening gesture embodies "viewing the sky."
- **Conflicting Ideas & Origins:**
  - Historicity of a single "Kōshōkun" is debated;
  - no primary proof he taught this exact form.

The name Kusanku is one of the most historically significant yet enigmatic in the karate canon, referring to a visiting Chinese martial arts master whose influence became foundational to Okinawan karate. The very first known written reference to an individual named Kusankun (or Koshokun) is found in the Oshima Hikki, a document compiled in 1762 by the Confucian scholar

Tobe Ryoen. This document recounts a shipwrecked Ryukyuan official's encounter with the martial arts master in 1756, noting a demonstration of grappling techniques. Crucially, the name was recorded in Katakana, as it was a foreign title or name unfamiliar to the Okinawan scribe.

While this is the earliest reference, the Chinese characters for his name/title are widely believed to have been 公相君, pronounced Koshokun in their native tongue, or Kusanku in Uchinaguchi. Though this is a modern adaptation rather than a traditional name, its meaning is key to understanding the figure. The first character, 公 (ko), translates to "public" or "official," highlighting a connection to state affairs. The second character, 相 (sho), means "minister" or "advisor," indicating a position of counsel and governance. The term concludes with 君 (kun), an honorific that conveys reverence, translating to "sir" or "master." Together, these characters embody the essence of a dignified figure in a position of public service and authority, suggesting the name was a formal rank rather than a personal name.

This original name underwent a significant philosophical reinterpretation by Gichin Funakoshi. In his effort to adapt karate for mainland Japanese audiences, Funakoshi renamed the kata Kanku ("gazing at the sky"). This change was an attempt to inject a more universal philosophical and aesthetic resonance into the form, moving away from a foreign-sounding title. Whether the name references a historical man or a metaphor, the kata ultimately became emblematic of the transmission of martial knowledge from China to Okinawa. Funakoshi's reinterpretation of the opening gesture—the practitioner looking upward—imbued the kata with new cultural significance, symbolizing modesty and philosophical aspiration.

Kusanku's Historical Origins

The origins of the kata are intrinsically linked to the Chinese martial artist known as Kusankun or Koshokun, who visited the Ryukyu Kingdom around 1756. His arrival coincided with a significant period of Chinese cultural and martial influence in Okinawa, particularly through diplomatic and scholarly exchanges in the mid-to-late 18th century. This timeline suggests that the kata's origins predate the Meiji-era Japanization of karate, indicating a relatively unaltered Sino-Okinawan lineage.

While the specifics of the master's life remain speculative, he is said to have demonstrated grappling techniques, including a distinctive scissor-leg takedown. His most notable student, Sakugawa Kangi, is widely believed to have formalized the kata as a tribute to his teacher. Sakugawa likely codified Kusanku both as a mnemonic tool for the techniques he learned and as a lasting homage to his respected mentor. Other figures may also be associated with the form, including Chatan Yara, who is thought to have contributed variations such as Chatan Yara no Kusanku.

The kata's unique combination of techniques is generally believed to reflect a fusion of Chinese White Crane boxing and other Quanfa traditions with indigenous Okinawan grappling and striking arts. Similar to the Pinan forms derived from Channan, Kusanku is likely a synthesis of these influences rather than a strict preservation of a single, unaltered style.

Exploring Kusanku's Wisdom

Kusanku showcases a wide variety of stances, often featuring dramatic transitions that emphasize evasiveness, changes in vertical levels, and spiraling momentum. Its key techniques include open-hand strikes and deflections, which effectively redirect attacks while delivering powerful counterattacks. In addition to these strikes, scissor kicks and leg entanglements are crucial for maintaining balance and controlling an opponent's movements, and evasive shifts allow for agile responses to incoming threats, enhancing the ability to evade and counterattack seamlessly.

Some schools interpret the kata as focusing on grappling, while others see it as emphasizing evasive striking. Moreover, some practitioners view it as incorporating techniques for night fighting that emphasize limb control and the art of off-balancing, providing a comprehensive approach to self-defense in various situations.

Kusanku's Diverse Paths

The rich history of Kusanku is marked by numerous versions that reflect its evolution through distinct lineages and educational objectives. One of the earliest forms is Sakugawa no Kusanku, attributed to Sakugawa Kanga (sometimes credited to his father, Sakugawa Kangi). The Chatan Yara no Kusanku is possibly even older and is preserved in various Tomari-based traditions. The art was significantly shaped by Anko Itosu, who developed the forms Kusanku Sho and Dai specifically for Okinawan schools, contributing to their widespread practice. Later, Gichin Funakoshi adapted these forms for Japan, renaming them Kanku and further influencing their development. The Shito-ryu variants are also noteworthy for their extensive range of interpretations, which include both Kusanku Sho and Dai, enriching the tapestry of this martial art.

These variations in style and form can be attributed to several key factors. First, pedagogical simplification, a concept promoted by Itosu, led to the restructuring of complex forms to improve understanding and accessibility for students. Additionally, Japanization and philosophical reframing, as seen in Funakoshi's work, played a significant role in adapting martial arts to resonate more deeply with Japanese culture and values. Furthermore, the artistic expansion contributed by masters like Mabuni integrated diverse stylistic elements and techniques, while the natural process of fragmented transmission over time also influenced how these practices are understood today. These differences are particularly evident in the divergent stylistic emphases between the Shuri and Tomari branches of karate. For example, Shotokan's Kanku-dai is a notably longer kata that emphasizes athleticism, while Shito-ryu is characterized by its broad range of interpretations, allowing for a wider exploration of techniques within its practice.

Kusanku's lasting influence extends beyond its direct lineages. Its evasive patterns and stance transitions were foundational, informing the design of later katas such as Gojushiho and the Pinan series. The kata's emphasis on tactical movement continues to serve as a template for many advanced forms. In addition to its technical legacy, the kata is surrounded by intriguing theories. Some suggest that Kusanku was specifically designed for night fighting, which would explain its reliance on tactile and low-visibility applications. The kata's iconic opening move, in which the practitioner gazes at the sky, has been interpreted both as a spiritual gesture symbolizing humility and philosophical aspiration, as well as a practical combative observation tactic.

Within the Matsumura Seito lineage, the Kusanku kata serves as a crucial historical touchstone, characterized by its direct and uninterrupted transmission. Unlike the Itosu-based traditions that split the form for teaching purposes, the version practiced here is a single, lengthy, and advanced kata. This form was passed down directly from Soken Hohan, through Kise Fusei to Kise Isao. This lineage, tracing its roots back to Matsumura Sokon, is believed to preserve a form that is closer to the original pre-Itosu adaptations, designed as a holistic fighting system rather than a segmented teaching tool.

This martial-centric identity is reinforced by the kata's technical focus on close-range tactics and grappling, which align directly with the historical legend of Kusanku's grappling demonstrations. The form features intricate and complex hand motions for trapping and limb control, low and evasive stances for off-balancing, and multi-layered applications, including joint locks, throws, and pressure point strikes hidden within its movements. Importantly, in this context, the symbolic interpretations of "night fighting" and "sky gazing" are absent. Instead, the kata represents a final, comprehensive test of mastery within the Kenshinkan curriculum, requiring practitioners to demonstrate a complete understanding of all the style's core principles.

Kusanku's Lasting Impact

Kusanku serves as both a historical artifact and a living practice, with its technical, symbolic, and pedagogical elements revealing the complex syncretism at the core of Okinawan karate. From Sakugawa's initial tribute to a Chinese master to Funakoshi's later philosophical reinterpretation, the kata maps the martial evolution of the archipelago across centuries.

Practicing Kusanku means engaging with a lineage that spans empires and ideologies. Although the Chinese envoy himself left little historical trace, the kata named after him has become a cornerstone of the art—not through rigid preservation, but through adaptive reinvention. Its iconic opening movement, in which practitioners look skyward, reminds us that even forgotten figures can cast long shadows, with their legacy living on through the movements they inspired.

Rohai

Okinawa's Heron Flow

Introduction to Rohai

Few kata exemplify the fragmentation of Okinawan martial transmission as clearly, or as contentiously, as Rohai. Today, what is recognized as Rohai across karate's major styles is less a unified form and more a series of interpretations that have only tenuous connections to one another. While Gojushiho splits into two or three recognizable branches, Rohai fragments completely: there is the Itosu-ha variant, often taught in the Shotokan tradition as Meikyo; the lesser-known Matsumora-ha version, preserved in a handful of Tomari-te-derived lineages; and numerous interpretations claimed by various offshoots, sometimes under different names or reinterpreted through a modern lens.

The term "Rohai" (鷺牌) translates roughly to "vision of a heron" or "crane stance/ form," and is often interpreted symbolically rather than literally. However, even this name is ambiguous. Some variants emphasize grace and posture, invoking the image of the crane, while others focus on sharp, linear strikes and explosive movements. Some associate Rohai with Tomari-te influences, others with Shuri-te, and some even suggest external origins from Chinese Quanfa.

This chapter will explore the diverse paths that the kata has taken, scrutinize the surviving forms, and challenge the notion that Rohai represents a single cohesive heritage. Rather than attempting to unify its fragments, we will examine what their divergence reveals about the development of Okinawan kata and the politics of inheritance.

Exploring Rohai's Essence

- **Traditional Notation:** 鷺牌 (common); alt. 老梅 appears historically in some lineages.
- **Script Breakdown:**
    - 鷺 "heron";
    - 牌 "tablet/insignia" (by extension "image/sign").
- **Core Meaning:** "Heron sign/figure."
- **Modern Interpretations:** Shotokan rename: 明鏡 (Meikyō, "bright mirror"), reframing the theme.
- **Conflicting Ideas & Origins:** Multiple Tomari/Itosu versions; kanji choice (鷺牌 vs. others) varies by lineage.

A cornerstone in several karate styles, Rohai boasts a rich history related to its name, origins, and evolution. Examining its etymology reveals a tapestry woven from Okinawan tradition, Chinese influence, and the impacts of significant figures who shaped the development of karate.

The traditional Okinawan name, Rohai (鷺牌), is often translated as "Vision of a Crane" or "Vision of a Heron." This name is thought to reflect the kata's unique movements, particularly the one-legged stance known as Sagi Ashi Dachi, which visually resembles a crane or heron at rest. The use of Kanji (鷺牌) in early Okinawan documents strengthens this interpretation, as the characters translate to "Heron Signboard" or "Vision of a Heron." Additionally, the name's meaning may have been influenced by White Crane Kung Fu traditions in Okinawa, as the Chinese pronunciation of Rohai (鷺牌) is "Lù pái."

However, the kata's identity changed significantly with Gichin Funakoshi. When he introduced it to mainland Japan, he renamed it Meikyo (明鏡), which means "bright mirror" or "mirror of the soul." This new name, likely inspired by the kata's opening technique where the practitioner pulls both palms up to the face, symbolized a philosophical shift. In Shotokan, the kata was reframed to emphasize spiritual refinement and self-reflection, creating a new legacy distinct from its Okinawan roots. This dual identity, the traditional Okinawan Rohai and the mainland Japanese Meikyo, illustrates the kata's adaptability and enduring legacy.

Exploring Rohai's Wisdom

Despite the significant differences found in its various forms, several mechanical themes consistently define the essence of Rohai across different lineages. All versions emphasize verticality and balance, with practitioners regularly challenging their core stability by transitioning between high and low stances. The kata's most prominent and recognizable feature is the one-legged stance, or crane pose. Although its execution and interpretation vary widely, this stance can serve as a test of balance, a deceptive feint, or a fluid transitional moment.

While linear strikes are present, Rohai generally characterized by off-angle attacks, circular motions, and deceptive rhythms. This is highlighted by a characteristic snap-and-pause rhythm that punctuates its explosive actions, resembling both White Crane and other Chinese martial arts styles. These movements often suggest sophisticated techniques, including throws and reaping actions concealed within the form, as well as grappling entries and close-range manipulations.

Ultimately, Rohai stands as a powerful example of how a kata can evolve from a martial archetype into a stylistic abstraction. Its fragmentation across different systems not only reflects the varying pedagogical goals of different masters but also the competing claims to lineage and authority. The resulting forms, though divergent, each provide a unique perspective into the martial systems that have preserved them.

Rohai's Historical Origins and Disputed Lineage

The kata known as Rohai is not a single, unified form but rather an archetypal framework of motion, posture, and balance that has been expressed differently over time and through various stylistic approaches. Its history is marked by competing and often unclear lineages, making it difficult to trace with certainty. The most widely accepted origin links Rohai to the Tomari-based teachings of Matsumora Kosaku (1829–1898), who is also credited with versions of Wanshu and Chinto. This connection suggests a foundation in the coastal village tradition that integrated

Chinese martial influences with native Okinawan fighting methods. However, no documentation from Matsumora himself exists to confirm this lineage, leaving it somewhat opaque.

Another lineage attributes one or more versions of Rohai to Itosu Anko (1831–1915), who is often recognized for modifying or codifying older forms for school instruction. Some oral traditions even suggest that Matsumura Sokon practiced Rohai, prehaps passing one or more on to Itosu, although, again, there is no direct evidence to support this claim.

These fragmented origins are exemplified by the differing forms preserved by two of karate's most influential masters: Mabuni Kenwa and Gichin Funakoshi.

Mabuni Kenwa's Shito-ryu system retains three distinct versions of Rohai, which he designated as Shodan, Nidan, and Sandan. The sequencing of these forms may reflect a pedagogical ordering rather than a historical one. Rohai Shodan is the closest in rhythm and posture to the version found in older Tomari-based schools, featuring balanced transitions between cat stance (neko-ashi dachi), crane stances, and snap-style strikes. In contrast, Rohai Nidan and Sandan introduce more elaborate movements, including unusual shifts in body level and off-angle strikes, suggesting either later additions or integrations from various sources. Some researchers speculate that Mabuni synthesized these forms from both the Matsumora and Itosu lineages or included material derived from Chinese-influenced forms that are no longer extant. Others believe they were teaching tools designed to create a progressive structure across the three forms.

Gichin Funakoshi's version of Rohai underwent significant changes when it transitioned to Shotokan, where it was renamed Meikyo (meaning "bright mirror"). This rebranding represents not just a new name but a profound conceptual shift, as Meikyo emphasizes fluidity and large, expressive movements over the sharp, short bursts characteristic of older Rohai forms. While the trademark crane-like balance on one leg remains, its purpose appears more aesthetic than combative. Some Shotokan practitioners view Meikyo as a kata of spiritual refinement rather than a tool for combat application; a mirror reflecting one's internal form rather than a means of achieving combat realism. Although the exact intent behind Meikyo is debatable, the divergence from the older Okinawan versions is evident, highlighting the significant impact of Japanization on Karate's forms.

While other traditions have struggled with the fragmented legacies of Rohai, the Matsumura Seito lineage has followed its own distinct path marked by intentional evolution. For many years, their curriculum included two Rohai kata, referred to as Rohai 1 and Rohai 2. The second kata, Rohai 2, was a Jodan version similar to the Matsumora Rohai, passed down through the teachings of Soken Hohan.

However, a significant restructuring of this tradition was later initiated by Kise Isao. In a decision reminiscent of Itosu's codification of other kata, Kise Sensei revived Rohai Chudan and Rohai Gedan. He drew from training notes and videos from Soken Hohan and his father, Kise Fusei. The objective was to align the curriculum with the oral traditions that Matsumura Sokon had originally practiced all three levels of Rohai. As a result of this change, the original Rohai 1 kata fell out of practice.

The newly established progression, Rohai Jodan, Rohai Chudan, and Rohai Gedan, was carefully designed to formalize and structure the teaching of Rohai for future generations. This approach ensures a systematic method for learning its unique postures, fluid transitions, and combative principles within the Matsumura Seito lineage.

Rohai's Lasting Impact

Rohai resists a single interpretation. Its many variations highlight the adaptable, sometimes chaotic transmission of Okinawan martial knowledge. While some may view this as a dilution of purity, others see it as a validation of adaptability. Regardless, Rohai, like the crane it is said to represent, remains poised delicately between stillness and motion, tradition and innovation, form and fragment.

Understanding Rohai does not require us to resolve its contradictions. Instead, we should recognize what its differences reveal about the evolution of kata, stylistic ambition, and the flexible identity of Okinawan martial arts.

WANSU
OKINAWA'S DRAGON THROW

Introduction to Wansu

In the rich and sprawling tapestry of Okinawan Karate kata, Wansu (ワンシュー or 汪楫) holds a particularly enigmatic and captivating position. Unlike some forms with well-documented origins, Wansu hints at ancient connections; its movements echo the profound influence of Chinese martial traditions that shaped the foundations of Ryukyuan fighting arts. At first glance, its techniques may seem perplexing or even counterintuitive, yet within its unique sequence lies a sophisticated combative logic.

This exploration will examine the origins of Wansu, the linguistic discussions surrounding its name, its distinctive technical contributions, and its lasting legacy as a tangible link to the ancient martial exchanges between Okinawa and China.

Exploring Wansu's Essence

- **Traditional Notation:** 汪輯 is common in Okinawan sources.
- **Script Breakdown:**
  - 汪 (surname Wang);
  - 輯 "collection/compilation."
- **Core Meaning:** "Wang's compilation/series," usually tied to the Qing envoy Wang Ji (汪楫).
- **Modern Interpretations:** Shotokan rename: 燕飛 (Empi "swallow flight"), focusing on aerial dynamics.
- **Conflicting Ideas & Origins:**
  - Whether the kata is by Wang Ji or memorializes him is debated;
  - multiple kanji attestations exist (腕秀 etc.).

The name "Wansu" serves as a key to understanding its origins and ignites a linguistic and historical discussion that highlights its deep ties to Chinese culture. While some popular interpretations suggest that "Wansu" refers to a generic "prince" or "king's hand," implying royal or noble roots, the most compelling and historically supported theory connects the term to a specific historical figure.

This theory suggests that the kata was either created by or named in honor of a Chinese envoy. When pronounced with an Okinawan accent, "Wansu" closely resembles "Wang Ji." This linguistic connection, along with historical records, adds significant weight to this interpretation, emphasizing the direct and personal transmission of martial knowledge.

Thus, the name reflects not just a vague concept, but rather a specific historical encounter, underscoring the deep cultural significance of a foreign master's visit and his lasting influence on Okinawa's martial heritage. It stands as a living artifact, a phonetic echo through the centuries, illustrating the profound cross-cultural exchange that characterizes Okinawan martial arts.

Wansu's Historical Origins

The genesis of Wansu is firmly rooted in a crucial period of Ryukyuan history, a time when cultural and martial exchanges with China were at their peak. The creation and transmission of this kata are inextricably linked to a specific, well-documented historical event.

The form is primarily associated with Wang Jí (汪楫), a high-ranking Chinese envoy who hailed from the costal region of Southern China known as the Fujian Province. Fujian was renowned for its sophisticated martial arts traditions, particularly its close-quarters combat systems and unique hand techniques. Wang Jí's background suggests he was not merely a diplomat but also a practitioner or patron of these formidable arts.

He is known to have led a significant diplomatic mission to Okinawa in 1683, as part of the ongoing tributary relationship between the Ryukyu Kingdom and the Ming/Qing Dynasties of China. This relationship fostered a continuous flow of cultural, intellectual, and martial knowledge.

The Chinese envoys, as representatives of a powerful and culturally advanced empire, often demonstrated their martial prowess during their visits to the Ryukyu Kingdom. These demonstrations were not merely for entertainment; they served as displays of cultural sophistication, military strength, and philosophical depth. It is highly probable that Wang Jí, or members of his skilled retinue, performed their martial arts during their stay, showcasing the techniques of their Fujianese heritage. It is from this significant encounter, whether through direct instruction, careful observation, or a combination thereof, that Okinawan martial artists absorbed and adapted the movements and principles that would later coalesce into the Wansu kata. This direct, person-to-person exchange underscores the profound impact of Chinese martial arts on early Okinawan Te.

The historical evidence for Chinese martial arts demonstrations in Okinawa provides a crucial context for understanding the transmission of these techniques. These exchanges were not isolated incidents but part of a continuous cultural dialogue that profoundly shaped the indigenous Okinawan fighting systems. While there isn't a single "lost" precursor form explicitly named for Wansu in the same way Channan is linked to Pinan, the kata embodies the spirit and techniques of the Southern Chinese styles that Wang Jí would have represented. It stands as a living testament to the deep martial connections forged across the East China Sea.

Applying Wansu's Wisdom

Wansu is particularly renowned for several distinctive techniques that highlight its unique approach to combat. Among these are the "Dumping" or "Dropping" Techniques, which stand out as some of the most recognizable elements of the kata. In certain versions of the form, the practitioner employs a controlled descent, seemingly collapsing their body weight with a subtle shift in balance. This technique is not about falling but rather about expertly unbalancing an opponent—using gravity to pull them off their feet or drive them to the ground. It skillfully demonstrates the principle of leveraging one's own weight to manipulate an opponent's structure.

Another hallmark of Wansu is the "Dragon Boy" Technique, characterized by its swift and often deceptive hand movements. This signature motion can serve multiple functions: it may deliver a lightning-fast strike to a vital point, act as a precise block to deflect incoming attacks, or facilitate subtle joint manipulations to control an opponent's limb. Its elusive nature makes it particularly challenging for opponents to defend against, as it relies on speed, precision, and a deep understanding of human anatomy.

Together, these techniques exemplify the distinctive lineage of Wansu, emphasizing close-quarters combat and the disruption of dynamic balance. The kata's bunkai reveals methods for seizing, throwing, and striking in rapid succession, showcasing a pragmatic self-defense approach that integrates various combative elements.

Although Wansu may not be typically associated with the overt internal cultivation seen in forms like Sanchin or Tensho, its focus on fluid transitions and the subtle manipulation of balance requires a sophisticated understanding of internal mechanics. The dynamic weight shifts and coordinated use of the entire body to generate power inherent in the "dropping" techniques necessitate a high degree of ki awareness and controlled relaxation. Likewise, the "dragon boy" techniques depend on focused kime (focus) and the efficient channeling of energy, illustrating that internal aspects are deeply woven into Wansu's combat framework, albeit expressed through a distinct physical vocabulary.

Wansu's Diverse Paths

The journey of Wansu through the centuries has seen its essence preserved across various Okinawan karate styles, with each lineage subtly adapting and interpreting the kata according to its own philosophical and technical priorities. This evolution reflects the dynamic nature of martial traditions, where forms are not static relics but living expressions that are passed down and refined by generations of masters.

The history of Wansu's transmission is a testament to its enduring value, and it has been passed down through prominent masters, including those who would later establish distinct styles. For instance, Wansu is a foundational kata in many Shorin-ryu lineages, reflecting its importance in the Shuri-te tradition that influenced masters such as Anko Itosu. It also made its way into Shito-ryu, founded by Kenwa Mabuni, who meticulously preserved and transmitted his version of the kata, thanks to his encyclopedic knowledge. Even within Isshin-ryu, a later composite style, a version of Wansu exists, demonstrating its pervasive influence across the landscape of Okinawan martial arts.

Significant stylistic variations of Wansu exist across these different schools and while the core sequence and signature techniques remain recognizable, the execution, emphasis, and even interpretation of bunkai can differ significantly. For example, some versions might emphasize a more direct and powerful approach to the "dumping" techniques, while others might focus on a more subtle off-balancing manipulation. The precise angles of the "dragon boy" hand movements and the body mechanics of the strong arm techniques can also vary, reflecting the unique teaching methods of each lineage.

The evolution of Wansu, therefore, mirrors the broader development of Okinawan karate itself, which is a constant process of adaptation and refinement.

Legends and anecdotes surrounding Wansu often focus on its mysterious origins and the powerful, almost supernatural, efficacy of its techniques. The tale of Wang Jí, a foreign master who shared his profound knowledge, is a legend in itself, underscoring the reverence with which these Chinese influences were received, and the enduring presence of this form's unique techniques in various lineages speaks volumes about its perceived effectiveness and the lasting fascination it holds for practitioners.

Wansu's Lasting Impact

All of this shows how Wansu is a profound and intriguing testament to the deep historical and martial connections between Okinawa and China. The name itself, which is the subject of ongoing debate, likely refers to the significant visit of Chinese envoy Wang Jí in 1683. This visit marked a pivotal moment of cultural exchange, enriching the development of Okinawan Te. Wansu is a living reflection of Fujianese Quanfa and embodies principles of close-quarters combat and dynamic balance manipulation, which continue to fascinate and challenge practitioners.

More than just a historical curiosity, Wansu is an essential part of the Okinawan Karate curriculum in various traditional styles. Its distinctive techniques, such as "dumping" and "dragon boy," provide a unique approach to self-defense, emphasizing finesse, timing, and internal power rather than sheer brute force. The variations found across different lineages highlight the adaptive nature of Okinawan martial arts, where core principles are preserved while being reinterpreted to fit specific teaching methods and combat philosophies.

Wansu serves as a powerful reminder of Karate's complex lineage. This martial tradition has consistently absorbed, adapted, and refined foreign influences to create its own unique and formidable identity. It remains a kata that whispers secrets of ancient exchanges, inviting practitioners to explore the rich, layered history of the "China Hand" that shaped Okinawa's martial essence.

WANDUAN

OKINAWA'S FLUID PATH

Introduction to Wanduan

At first glance, Wanduan may seem like a sibling to Kanshiwa, and in many ways, it is. Both were created by Uechi Kanei, both reflect his commitment to structured pedagogy, and both serve as transitional forms, guiding students from the rigid Sanchin into the flowing complexity of advanced kata. However, Wanduan is much more than just a "next step." It is a refined expression of the Uechi-ryu lineage, rich in symbolism, influenced by Chinese martial traditions, and connected to deeper Okinawan oral traditions.

Despite being relatively recent in its creation, Wanduan carries significant conceptual weight, both as a tribute to the founders and in its potential etymological roots tracing back to ancient Chinese systems. This chapter explores the kata's origins, meaning, practical structure, and its place within the broader context of Okinawan martial development. It challenges us to view modern kata not as mere modernizations but as evolving encapsulations of ancient lessons.

Exploring the Essence of Wanduan

- **Traditional Notation**: Katakana—ワンダン.
- **Script Breakdown**: Spelled "W-A-N-D-U-A-N" in Japanese phonetics; not rendered in kanji, indicating foreign or phonetic origin.
- **Core Meaning**: Modern interpretations often render it as "King's Road" or "Way of the King", derived from Chinese wáng dào ("king's path")—a metaphor for royal lineage or martial sovereignty.
- **Modern Interpretations**: Commonly linked to prestige and martial mastery, sometimes interpreted as representing a "royal" form taught sparingly to advanced practitioners. ("Head of state" metaphor in forum commentary)
- **Conflicting Ideas & Origins:**
  - Chinese origin theory: Suggests linkage to northern Chinese kung-fu nomenclature and Royal guard techniques.
  - Okinawan legend theory: Associates the form with mbedment in Okinawan royal lineage, especially the king's personal guard.
  - Disputed authenticity: Some consider Wanduan a modern invention or an esoteric kata with uncertain provenance, not found in standard curricula.

The name Wanduan (完段) holds multiple interpretations, both linguistic and symbolic. In Uechi-ryu circles, it is a tribute to the founders Uechi Kanbun and Shushiwa. This lineage naming combines "Kan" (完) and "Wa" (和), connecting the kata directly to these pivotal figures in the system. Some traditions write the name as 完段, where "dan" (段) can signify level or rank, suggesting a path of progression or a stepping stone in martial arts.

Another, less widely accepted theory links Wanduan to a Chinese form known as Kang Zang Tzou, often translated as "Emperor's War Hands." This association gives rise to the nickname "King's Road," which refers to a metaphorical journey of disciplined training, noble bearing, and philosophical direction. If this translation holds true, it endows the kata with a deeper sense of purpose: serving as a journey of principled conflict resolution and personal sovereignty.

There is ongoing debate within specific martial arts communities about whether Wanduan should be categorized as an original Okinawan kata or a reconstruction based on lost Chinese forms. What remains clear, however, is that its name, regardless of the kanji used, symbolizes both homage and aspiration. Whether it represents legacy or the "King's Path," Wanduan encourages practitioners to embody mastery and respect.

Wanduan's Historical Origins

Wanduan, like Kanshiwa, was developed in 1954 by Uechi Kanei during a time when Okinawan karate was evolving from a secretive family practice into a public and more systematic discipline.

Kanei faced a significant teaching challenge: guiding modern students from the static, breath-centered Sanchin form to the more dynamic and nuanced Seisan and Sanseiryu. Wanduan emerged as a solution, designed to bridge the gap between conceptual understanding and practical application. It builds directly on Kanshiwa, while introducing more technical complexity, greater directional changes, and deeper application possibilities.

Although Kanei created Wanduan, he did so within the framework of his father, Uechi Kanbun's teachings, as well as the Chinese martial foundations passed down from Shushiwa. The movements in this kata closely resemble those found in Southern Chinese martial arts, specifically elements of Praying Mantis and White Crane, which emphasize trapping, redirection, and low, stable stances.

There is a persistent, though less substantiated, theory that connects Wanduan to the enigmatic figure Annan (Ahnan), a Chinese martial artist rumored to have taught in Okinawa during the 19th century. Whether this connection is historical or folkloric, it suggests that Wanduan may reflect older Chinese martial templates that have been lost to time but are remembered in fragments.

It should be noted that Wanduan has also been linked to the Oyadamari family lineage, which connects it to Tomari-te traditions. While Uechi-ryu is generally associated with Naha-te, this relationship highlights the interconnected and fluid nature of Okinawa's martial landscape.

Applying Wanduan's Wisdom

At its core, Wanduan is a refinement kata that adds complexity to the foundation established by Kanshiwa, enhancing a student's understanding of timing, mechanics, and internal coordination. It introduces a wider application of classical Uechi-ryu stances, emphasizing subtle shifts that challenge a student's ability to root themselves and adapt. Stability becomes a central theme, especially during transitional movements.

In terms of body mechanics, there is a strong focus on controlled redirection. Students are encouraged to transition smoothly between offensive and defensive postures while maintaining internal pressure and a sense of connection throughout their movements. Key techniques become more sophisticated, particularly the Circular Blocks, which evolve beyond the basic mechanics of Kanshiwa into more reactive applications. Trapping motions play a crucial role in these transitional sequences, allowing practitioners to interpret their movements as either joint control or limb clearance. Continuing the Uechi tradition, techniques such as Elbow Strikes and Palm-Heel Thrusts are emphasized, focusing on close-range, bone-targeted impacts. Kicks are also an essential element, reinforcing balance in motion through chambered snapping kicks directed at the midline.

While the focus on breath and internal timing is less pronounced than in Sanchin, Wanduan still requires students to be mindful of their breath timing and internal focus. Movements should feel grounded yet fluid, embodying an essence that feels alive rather than robotic. Overall, the kata challenges students to coordinate motion, breathing, focus, and posture into a cohesive combative form. For advanced practitioners, Wanduan offers endless potential for refinement; each repetition revealing new mechanical inefficiencies to address.

The bunkai of Wanduan, often taught in a linear fashion, is actually adaptable and multidirectional, likely reflecting its Southern Chinese roots. The kata begins with initial engagements that focus on intercepting or redirecting movements, which are particularly effective for countering linear strikes or grabs. As the practitioner progresses, they encounter several transitions that can be interpreted as wrist entrapments or tuite applications, enabling effective control of the opponent's upper body. In terms of offensive techniques, low-line kicks and snapping strikes are incorporated to disrupt balance or target the legs and midsection; characteristic elements of Uechi-ryu's close-range engagement. The kata also features sequences that emphasize elbow-hip coordination, linking to techniques for breaking away from clinches or disrupting an opponent's structure. Furthermore, the integration of pressure points is evident, as several strikes align with traditional kyusho targets, reinforcing Uechi-ryu's combative logic rooted in Chinese medicine.

Ultimately, Wanduan teaches control: of oneself, one's breath, the surrounding space, and the opponent. Its layered nature makes it a reliable testing ground for analyzing not only technique but also mindset under pressure.

Wanduan's Diverse Path

Wanduan was developed during the modern period and is closely associated with the Uechi-ryu system. Similar to its counterpart, Kanshiwa, it has experienced less stylistic fragmentation than older katas. However, minor variations exist across different dojos and affiliated styles.

Koburyu includes Wanduan in its curriculum, preserving the original structural intent while allowing for varying interpretations of some applications. Additionally, some schools use different naming conventions or refer to the kata by its historical form or an alternate lineage variant. Notably, adaptations for youth or public education often simplify specific movements, reflecting an Okinawan trend of customizing katas for teaching purposes. These adaptations aim to maintain the core principles of the kata while making it more accessible to learners.

Importantly, because Wanduan originated from Uechi Kanei's standardization efforts, it embodies a unique moment of purpose-built pedagogy. It is a modern kata that has not been diluted by decades of informal transmission but has been carefully crafted with clarity in mind.

Wanduan's Lasting Impact

Wanduan may not have ancient roots, but it embodies the weight of tradition in every detail. This kata is a deliberate fusion of legacy and evolution, created not out of necessity, but with intent. By connecting Kanshiwa and the more advanced Uechi forms, it allows practitioners to navigate a crucial stage of development.

Its name, whether interpreted as a tribute to Kanbun and Shushiwa or as the "King's Road," reflects a kata that possesses depth and purpose. Wanduan demands control, not only of one's limbs but also of one's intention. It rewards precision and punishes disconnection.

In the ever-evolving landscape of Okinawan karate, Wanduan remains a steadfast guide. It teaches not just movement, but movement with meaning.

ANANKU

OKINAWA'S EFFICIENT STRIKES

Introduction to Ananku

Often overshadowed by more widely practiced kata, Ananku holds a unique position within the Tomari-te lineage and the broader context of Okinawan Karate. This kata is frequently described as elegant, direct, and deceptively simple. It stands out for its unusual transitions, compact structure, and the balanced use of both open-hand and closed-hand techniques, however, its origins remain a topic of ongoing debate.

Ananku is believed to have been either created or popularized by Kyan Chotoku in the early 20th century. Some sources attribute its development to Kyan's tenure at the Kadena Agricultural School around 1931, possibly as part of an effort to integrate Karate into the public education system, while others suggest that older oral traditions link it to a mysterious Chinese martial artist known only as "Anan," whose shipwreck in Tomari is said to have influenced the kata's structure.

This chapter will explore the contested origins of Ananku, its distinctive techniques, and its cultural and curricular significance. We will investigate the kata's linguistic roots, dissect its core applications, and assess its place within the evolution of Tomari-te and Okinawan martial arts as a whole.

Exploring Ananku's Essence

- **Traditional Notation:** Competing: 安南光 ("southern light"); 安南空 ("southern sky"); 安南公 ("lord Annan"); also アーナンクー.
- **Script Breakdown:**
  - 安南 "Annan" (historical term for Vietnam/south).
  - 光 "light"; 空 "sky/void";
  - 公 "lord."
- **Core Meaning:** Popularly "Light/Peace from the South."
- **Modern Interpretations:** Linked to Kyan Chōtoku's Taiwan trip or to a teacher, "Annan."
- **Conflicting Ideas & Origins:** No single authoritative kanji; schools adopt different spellings to reflect their oral history.

The name Ananku (安南光), commonly translated as "Light from the South" or "Peaceful Southern Light," can be interpreted both literally and symbolically. Some believe it refers to the kata's supposed Taiwanese origin, while others suggest it metaphorically represents enlightenment, guidance, or philosophical illumination from the south.

However, according to some oral traditions, a Fujianese sailor or martial artist named Anan is said to have taught the techniques that inspired the kata after surviving a shipwreck near Tomari. If this account is accurate, the name might serve as a homage rather than merely a descriptive term.

This ambiguity adds to the kata's mystique and highlights the blending of myth, oral history, and symbolism often found in Okinawan martial traditions.

Ananku's Historical Origins

Kyan Chotoku is primarily credited with introducing or even developing the kata Ananku. His style combined agility with precision, highlighting quick directional changes, light footwork, and deceptive simplicity; all of which are evident in Ananku.

We know that Kyan taught karate at the Kadena Agricultural School in the early 1930s, and some sources claim that he created Ananku specifically for his students there. If this is true, the kata would have emerged during a time of increasing standardization and public dissemination of martial arts within the school system. However, other accounts attribute the kata's origin to the earlier influence of the aforementioned mysterious figure named "Anan," whom Kyan is said to have met.

Regardless of whether it was developed or adapted, Ananku served two purposes: as an instructional kata for novice to intermediate students and as a means of preserving the distinct elements of Tomari-te, separate from Shuri-te and Naha-te. Its concise structure and clarity make it particularly useful for developing directional transitions and coordination.

If the story of Anan holds any truth, the kata may also reflect southern Chinese martial principles, especially in its open-hand techniques and compact, reactive posture. Comparisons have been made to the White Crane or Southern Shaolin systems. Nonetheless, its core structure seems heavily influenced by Tomari-te traditions, particularly those passed down by Matsumora and Kyan.

Applying Ananku's Wisdom

Ananku is a kata characterized by its clean, angular techniques and emphasis on quick changes in direction, fostering spatial awareness and dynamic control through short bursts of power rather than lengthy combinations. Its signature movements prominently feature a down-block followed by a reverse punch, a fundamental staple across various martial styles, while also incorporating adaptable transitions into open-hand guarding postures.

Central to Ananku's unique approach are its stances and intricate footwork. The front stance provides a strong foundation for direct, linear engagement, while the horse stance offers crucial lateral stability for maintaining balance and control during movements. The cat stance, in turn, enhances transitional agility, enabling swift shifts in position and readiness. Complementing these stances, practitioners engage in shifting footwork paired with quick punches or palm-heel strikes, allowing for rapid offense and defense. Furthermore, high-to-low shifts in posture subtly suggest potential counters against grabs, throws, or takedowns, enhancing the fluidity and versatility of responses in combat.

The interpretation of Ananku's bunkai, or application of techniques, varies widely among different schools. Some practitioners view the kata's movements as straightforward linear and direct striking drills, while others interpret them as sophisticated entries into grappling or joint manipulation strategies. Elements such as open-hand techniques and body turns may also serve to obscure underlying sweeps, escapes, or redirection methods, offering a broad scope of practical application for those who delve deeper.

While Ananku may not emphasize breath control to the same overt extent as a kata like Sanchin, it nonetheless cultivates a vital coordination between breath, timing, and motion. Its practice powerfully reinforces kime alongside a heightened awareness of transitions, and in certain traditions, Ananku is also instrumental in cultivating the principle of muchimi, or sticky, flowing energy, all contained within a framework of compact, efficient motion.

Ananku's Diverse Paths

Ananku is a kata most prominently preserved in styles such as Shudokan, Matsubayashi-ryu, and several systems influenced by Tomari. Each of these styles has adapted or retained the form based on their specific teaching goals, resulting in variations in its execution. Some versions emphasize elongated stances and powerful strikes, while others prioritize speed and subtlety, as seen in Matsubayashi-ryu's tighter and more compact interpretation, which aligns with Kyan's emphasis on economy of motion.

These stylistic adaptations likely arise from the need to tailor the kata to different educational objectives. For instance, university-based systems might focus on larger movements for clarity and exercise, whereas traditional dojos tend to maintain a more compact and combative approach. Although Ananku has not directly led to derivative kata in the same way that Pinan or Gekisai have, its significant influence is evident in the technical progression of systems derived from Tomari-te.

Ananku's Lasting Impact

Ananku is not just a bridge kata or a regional curiosity; it represents a significant period in the development of Okinawan Karate by blending folklore, teaching methods, and combat insights. Whether it originated from Kyan's creativity or was influenced by a shipwrecked stranger, it embodies the Okinawan spirit of integration and evolution. Its concise elegance continues to provide valuable lessons in movement, awareness, and adaptability for today's martial artists.

WANKAN

OKINAWA'S ROYAL DEFENSE

Introduction to Wankan

Wankan may be the shortest kata in the Shotokan syllabus, but its brevity conceals a profound mystery and subtle sophistication. Its origins, creator, and early use remain uncertain, causing Wankan to often be overshadowed by more famous forms. However, in its flowing movements, strategic finesse, and meaningful name, it stands as a crown jewel of the Tomari-te tradition.

As a compact form with a regal essence, Wankan is characterized by a unique fusion of defense and offense into seamless motion. Although relatively obscure compared to foundational kata, Wankan is practiced in several major styles, including Shotokan, Shito-ryu, and Matsubayashi-ryu. Its Tomari-te roots give it a distinct flavor compared to Naha-te or Shuri-te derived forms, offering practitioners a brief yet powerful study in rhythm, timing, and control.

This chapter will explore Wankan not merely as a kata but as a strategic framework born from Okinawa's Tomari region. We will investigate its enigmatic name, trace its lineage, analyze its applications, and argue for its deeper significance as a kata that embodies symbolism and adaptability in the evolving world of Okinawan martial traditions.

Exploring Wankan's Essence

- **Traditional Notation:** 王冠 (Wankan).
- **Script Breakdown:**
  - 王 "king";
  - 冠 "crown."
- **Core Meaning:** "King's crown."
- **Modern Interpretations:** Shotokan lore links opening shape to a "crown"; other names (Shōfū, Hito) appear in literature.
- **Conflicting Ideas & Origins:** Attributions to Tomari lines are common; the exact origin of the title is unclear.

The name "Wankan," which means "King's Crown" in Chinese characters, is derived from the symbols for "King" (王) and "Crown" (冠). Throughout history, this kata has also been referred to by alternate names such as Okan, Shofu, which translates to "Pine Wind" (松風), and Matsukaze, another reading of the same characters.

There has been much linguistic and historical debate regarding the exact origin of the name "Wankan." One interpretation suggests that it symbolizes the kata's strategic superiority; the idea of a "crown" technique emphasizes refined control and finishing skill. Furthermore, some researchers point out that the term "Wan" represents an Okinawan reading that has been retained, as opposed to being Japanized like many other kata. This indicates that "Wankan" may have been included early in the kata's history and reflects its non-standardized transmission.

The use of alternate names such as "Pine Wind" implies a connection to an older poetic naming tradition, where imagery was evoked rather than strictly technical descriptions provided. The cultural significance of the name can be viewed through a symbolic lens, where the "King's Crown" embodies victory achieved not through sheer force but through superior positioning and composure. Additionally, it may reference the elegant circular techniques and sweeping arm movements associated with the kata, which exhibit a regal quality in both execution and demeanor. In this regard, Wankan becomes a metaphor for grace in combat, highlighting the beauty and strategy inherent in martial arts.

Wankan's Historical Origins

The origins of Wankan are shrouded in mystery, and its creator remains unknown. Unlike other kata with documented lineages, there are no records of who introduced or spread this form in Okinawa; it seems to have always been an integral part of the Tomari-te tradition. Shoshin Nagamine, a significant figure in documenting this lineage, notes that the kata was developed by an ancient master, whose name has unfortunately been lost to time. It is believed to have emerged in the mid-to-late 19th century within the martial circles of Tomari village. Its minimalist structure likely reflects the practical and efficient approach to combat refined by Tomari's warrior class. The kata appears to have been designed for rapid response, making it ideal for close-quarters and pragmatic engagement.

Applying Wankan's Wisdom

As a Tomari-te kata, Wankan shares a kinship with other compact, elusive forms like Wanshu and Rohai. Its flowing techniques and compound motions suggest a strong influence from Chinese martial forms that emphasize redirection, interception, and tactile control, the study of which leads it's practitioners to find a rich tapestry of techniques that emphasize balance, readiness, and fluidity.

One of the foundational elements is the cat stance, which provides stability while allowing for quick redirection of movement. As one moves through the kata, the walking footwork consists of slow, deliberate steps that hint at stealth, evoking a sense of slippery footing that could aid in evasion. Moreover, the kata features unfixed stances, where certain movements defy traditional constraints, resulting in a fluid and organic execution that feels natural.

Key techniques within Wankan include Hasami-uke, or the scissor block, which serves to trap or redirect incoming attacks, demonstrating a principle of control over the opponent's movements. The Koko-tsuki and Sukui-uke, both known as the tiger mouth techniques, one a scooping block and the other a thrust, illustrate concepts of entry control and joint manipulation. The Yama-tsuki, or mountain punch, serves as a powerful and symbolic dual strike that showcases the kata's dynamic energy.

As practitioners delve deeper, techniques like Morote sukui-uke highlight the importance of body unification and tension, often interpreted as a defense against kicks. The kata also incorporates Gyaku shuto-uke, tettsui-uchi, and mae-geri, which emphasize a blend of deflection and counterattacks, reinforcing the idea of disruption in combat situations.

In terms of applications, or bunkai, Wankan reveals insights into yielding to control. The techniques prioritize evasion and the ability to manage the direction of an attack. The close-range combat tactics promoted within the kata highlight strategies for operating at minimal distances, including clinches and redirection maneuvers. Additionally, modern interpretations of Wankan apply its principles to knife defense scenarios, showcasing the adaptability and relevance of these ancient techniques in contemporary martial arts practice.

Wankan's Diverse Paths

The Transmission History of the kata Wankan reveals its preservation in Tomari-te, from which it was passed down through various styles, including Shorin-ryu, Shito-ryu, Shotokan, Genseiryu, and Matsubayashi-ryu.

The incorporation of Wankan into styles such as Shotokan occurred much later during the modernization and codification of karate in the early to mid-20th century, likely in the 1930s or 1940s. While the connection to Wankan remains somewhat speculative, Yoshitaka Funakoshi is occasionally mentioned as a possible figure who may have influenced the version practiced today in Shotokan. This Shotokan modernization, which aimed to streamline kata, may have contributed to an abstraction of Wankan from its Tomari roots. In more contemporary times, Kancho Takemasa Okuyama has added his own interpretations and applications of the kata, especially focusing on knife defense, which has enriched Wankan's evolving legacy.

In contrast, styles like Shito-ryu and Matsubayashi-ryu maintain a closer relationship with the original Tomari flavor. The variations in Wankan can largely be attributed to the absence of a clear creator or central lineage, leading to different interpretations over time. Although Wankan has remained somewhat isolated and less influential compared to other katas, it offers unique insights into Tomari's approach to speed, flow, and practicality.

Wankan's Lasting Impact

Wankan, though brief in structure, encapsulates a strategic and poetic approach to combat. Its combination of evasion, redirection, and flowing counterstrikes makes it a hidden gem among the Tomari-te kata. While its lineage is shrouded in mystery and its techniques are subtle, its role as a study in adaptability and restraint is clear.

Often overlooked, Wankan continues to challenge advanced practitioners with its demand for precise timing, fluid control, and a nuanced understanding of movement. It serves not as a culmination but rather as a quiet apex—a reminder that in martial arts, depth often resides in simplicity, and the true mastery is achieved by those who embrace quiet efficiency.

SAIFA

OKINAWA'S CIRCULAR FORCE

Introduction to Saifa

Saifa is not characterized by elegance. It doesn't flow like a crane or roar like a tiger; instead, it crashes in, grabs, rips, and breaks. To the untrained eye, Saifa may seem almost crude, but beneath the sudden hammerfists and snapping joint controls lies a kata designed with clinical precision for real-world survival. As the first "real" kata that many students encounter after basic drills in various Goju-ryu systems, Saifa serves as a litmus test for the student's transition from foundational techniques to combative application. It introduces practitioners to circular energy, folding power, and aggressive disruption, all while reinforcing essential postures, directional changes, and controlled breathing.

This chapter delves into Saifa's dual nature: its brutal, close-range techniques and its elegant internal logic. With uncertain historical origins in Southern China, Saifa occupies a vital place at the beginning of Goju-ryu's classical kata, bridging explosive movements with efficient techniques and offering a glimpse into the survival-focused roots of Okinawan martial arts.

Exploring Saifa's Essence

- **Traditional Notation:** 砕破 (Saifa).
- **Script Breakdown:**
    - 砕 "smash/shatter";
    - 破 "break/rupture."
- **Core Meaning:** "Smash and break."
- **Modern Interpretations:** Goju frames force-disruption tactics under this title.
- **Conflicting Ideas & Origins:** Title is stable; meaning is literal; (general Goju lists corroborate kanji).

Saifa (砕破) is a term that is often translated as "Smash and Tear" or "Pound and Pulverize." The first character, 砕 (Sai), means to smash, shatter, or break, while the second character, 破 (Ha/Fa), signifies to tear, destroy, or rip apart. It's interesting to note that while the second character is pronounced "Ha" in standard Japanese, it is rendered as "Fa" in the Okinawan dialect. This distinction reflects a unique aspect of Okinawan phonetics and suggests a preservation of certain Chinese linguistic roots in the region.

Unlike poetic kata names referencing animals, winds, or mythical battles, Saifa is blunt and direct. It evokes immediate violence, not abstract spirituality. It describes what the kata does, not what it symbolizes. This lack of metaphor reflects the pragmatism of early Okinawan combat forms and suggests a purpose-driven design aligned with close-quarters self-defense.

Saifa's Historical Origins

The origins of the Saifa kata are rooted in the martial arts traditions of Southern China and its journey to Okinawa is defined by two key figures. Kanryo Higaonna (1853–1916) is traditionally recognized for introducing the form to Okinawa, drawing from his studies in Fuzhou. However, an interesting historical debate suggests that his student, Chojun Miyagi, who lived from 1888 to 1953, played a more significant role in developing or codifying Saifa as part of his broader systematization of Naha-te into Goju-ryu. This idea is supported by the fact that another prominent Higaonna student, Juhatsu Kyoda, did not incorporate Saifa into his To'on-ryu teachings, which lends weight to the theory of Miyagi's authorship. Consequently, the kata's creation period is uncertain; if it originated with Higaonna, it would date to the late 19th century, but if Miyagi authored it, its formalization would fall in the early 20th century.

Saifa's martial influences are clearly of Southern Chinese origin. It draws heavily from Kempo styles, with Akio Kinjo and other scholars highlighting suggestions of White Crane and possibly Lion-style boxing. While no direct precursor kata linking the form to others like the Anan form in Ryuei-ryu has been confirmed, it is likely that Saifa was born from a combination of fragmented drills and forms that either Higaonna or Miyagi encountered during their training in Fujian Province.

Crafted as an early, yet essential, kata, Saifa serves multiple purposes for the practitioner. It is designed to train explosive power and rapid directional changes, which are skills crucial for close-quarter combat. The form also helps practitioners develop effective counters to grabs and holds, offering practical applications in real-life situations. Through its practice, students are introduced to the unique dynamics of Goju, exploring the balance between hard and soft techniques as well as linear and circular movements. Ultimately, Saifa conditions the body to facilitate a seamless transition between offensive and defensive postures, thereby enhancing overall versatility in martial arts.

Applying Saifa's Wisdom

Saifa is a comprehensive study of foundational stances and tactical movement. The kata incorporates several key postures, including Shiko Dachi (Square Stance) to enhance rooted power, Neko Ashi Dachi (Cat Stance) for quick shifting and off-line evasion, and Sagi Ashi Dachi (Crane Stance) to maintain transitional balance and targeting. The overall movement involves a constant shift off the centerline, facilitating evasion and enabling simultaneous counter-attacks; its aggressive and short embusen closely mimicking the dynamics of real confrontations.

The kata's range of key techniques and bunkai is centered on effective close-range engagement. The Hasami-uke (Scissor Block) serves as a fundamental tool for trapping and redirecting incoming strikes. Likewise, close-range percussive strikes, such as Ura Uchi (Backfist) and Tettsui (Hammerfist), are designed to incapacitate an opponent. The versatile descending hammerfist, for instance, can be interpreted across different lineages as either a strike to the skull or a technique aimed at breaking the clavicle. Offensive tactics also include Mae Geri and Hiza

Geri, which target vulnerable areas like the groin, abdomen, or knee. The Morote Sukui-uke (Double-hand Scooping Block) exemplifies the kata's multifunctional approach, serving as a grip break, a limb trap, or even a takedown, adding tuite elements that involve wrist manipulations and joint redirections to be seamlessly integrated into transitions, especially after grip releases, adding a crucial layer of depth to the practitioner's skill set.

Saifa's Diverse Paths

The transmission history of Saifa highlights its evolution through several prominent karate systems, with Goju-ryu serving as its primary custodian. The kata was preserved and disseminated through Chojun Miyagi's curriculum but also spread to other schools. Notably, Shito-ryu adopted Saifa under Kenwa Mabuni, who bridged key lineages after training with both Higaonna and Itosu. Additionally, Saifa found its way into Kyokushin Karate through Mas Oyama, influenced by Goju elements from Nei-Chu So, a student of Gogen Yamaguchi.

Interestingly, Saifa is absent from Juhatsu Kyoda's To'on-ryu curriculum, supporting the theory that Miyagi formalized the kata after his training with Higaonna. Some Okinawan instructors suggest that the kata was originally taught without a formal name, acquiring its identity only when Miyagi began standardizing kata for the modern era.

These lineages have resulted in significant stylistic variations in how Saifa is practiced. In Japanese Goju, for instance, the descending hammerfist may differ in trajectory, and some lineages implement tighter stance transitions compared to their Okinawan counterparts. In Shito-ryu, additional flow and posture transitions are often incorporated, reflecting Mabuni's extensive cross-training. In contrast, Kyokushin tends to emphasize a more linear execution, focusing on impact power rather than fluid redirection. These variations can be attributed to various factors, including pedagogical evolution across different dojos, post-WWII adaptations, and the influence of Japanization and sportification on karate as a whole.

Saifa's impact extends beyond its own performance, as it serves as a crucial foundational form for other kata. Its close-in strategies and simplified bunkai structures provide a blueprint for the Gekisai kata, preparing students for the explosive techniques that follow and paving the way for more advanced circular manipulation kata. Throughout its journey, Saifa has remained a vital training tool, carrying forward a legacy of adaptability

Saifa's Lasting Impact

Saifa embodies the immediacy and grit of early Okinawan martial arts. It is explosive, efficient, and designed for survival when one is grabbed or cornered. Whether the kata was passed down from Chinese systems or developed by Miyagi himself, its essence lies in disrupting, breaking, and countering at close range.

As the first classical kata in the Goju-ryu system, Saifa continues to challenge new generations of karateka to engage in close combat, strike hard, and think quickly. Its true value isn't in its aesthetic appeal but in how effectively it teaches the body to move with force and purpose.

Saifa is a kata that attacks aggressively, dismantles defenses, and leaves a lasting impact on opponents and practitioners alike.

Shisochin
Okinawa's Open-Hand Tactics

Introduction to Shisochin

Few kata embody the paradox of power and subtlety quite like Shisochin. It moves with calm confidence, yet it explodes with focused ferocity. Shisochin is graceful but unrelenting; it expresses internal balance while masking the deadly intent below the surface. Although it may lack the notoriety of Suparinpei or the popularity of Seisan, Shisochin has earned a quietly revered place among Okinawan practitioners.

For Chojun Miyagi, the founder of Goju-ryu, this kata was not just another form in the curriculum; it was his favorite in his later years. Why? Perhaps because it combines hardness and softness, strategy and visceral action, in a way that few others can. Or perhaps it represented a maturity of technique: compact, efficient, and brutally effective.

This chapter explores Shisochin in depth, covering its etymology, symbolic overtones, Chinese roots, combat logic, and its place in the evolving martial tapestry of Okinawa. While Seisan embodies the strength of direct confrontation, Shisochin represents the strength of adaptability: quietly poised and ready to engage from any direction.

Exploring the Essence of Shisochin

- **Traditional Notation:** 四向鎮 (Shisōchin/Shisochin).
- **Script Breakdown:**
  - 四 "four";
  - 向 "directions";
  - 鎮 "to suppress/settle."
- **Core Meaning:** "Suppressing in four directions."
- **Modern Interpretations:** Read tactically as four-direction control.
- **Conflicting Ideas & Origins:** Stable in Goju nomenclature; exact original Fujian reading is debated.

Shisochin (四向戦) is commonly translated as "Four Directions of Conflict" or "Subduing the Four Directions." Each character in the term has a specific meaning. The first character, 四 (shi), means "four," which indicates a fundamental aspect of structure or numerology. The second character, 向 (so), translates to "direction" or "facing," suggesting movement or orientation. Lastly, the character 戦 (chin or sen) represents "war," "battle," or "conflict," evoking themes of struggle and confrontation. Together, these characters create a narrative that reflects the complexities of navigating conflict.

The name Shisochin conveys the idea of being surrounded or attacked from all sides, serving as a metaphor for combat and the unpredictable struggles of life. There is also a speculative connection to Sochin (壮鎮), another kata found in the Shotokan and Shito-ryu lineages. Some oral traditions suggest that Shisochin may have originally been named Sochin, with changes in characters and pronunciation demonstrating Okinawa's tendency to adapt and reinterpret kata influenced by Chinese traditions. Whether this represents a renaming of the same form or evidence of a shared origin remains uncertain.

The concept of "four directions" carries rich symbolic significance that can be explored in various ways. First, it evokes the four classical compass directions, representing not only spatial awareness but also a form of defense against challenges coming from any angle. This idea emphasizes the importance of understanding one's environment and being prepared to address threats from all sides. Additionally, it resonates with the four elements of traditional Chinese medicine: wood, fire, metal, and water. In this context, the fifth element, earth, symbolizes the practitioner who stands at the center, embodying a balance among these forces. Furthermore, this concept highlights the simultaneous cultivation of diverse strengths, both hard and soft, internal and external, mental and physical. This holistic approach underscores the significance of nurturing various aspects of oneself to achieve harmony and resilience.

Shisochin's Historical Origins

A kata of Chinese origin, Shisochin is closely associated with the Southern Shaolin styles taught in Fuzhou. These styles particularly emphasize open-hand striking, close-quarters manipulation, and a blend of Tiger and Crane principles.

The introduction of Shisochin to Okinawa is attributed to Kanryo Higaonna, the founder of Naha-te. Higaonna studied in Fuzhou under Chinese martial artists, including Ryu Ryu Ko, among others whose identities are not well-documented. Upon his return to Okinawa, Higaonna passed this kata on to his students, most notably Chojun Miyagi, who preserved and taught Shisochin as a core part of what became Goju-ryu.

While historical records do not provide an exact date for the formalization of the kata in Okinawa, it likely entered the local martial vocabulary in the late 19th century, during a period of increasing cultural exchange between Ryukyu and southern China. Shisochin arrived not as a standardized form, but as a living template; a set of combative principles expressed through movement. It was later formalized and refined by Miyagi and his successors. Unlike the school-drilled Pinan or the layered battlefield kata such as Passai, Shisochin appears to have been preserved for those already familiar with the internal logic of close-quarters combat. It was not intended for mass instruction, but rather for the transmission of nuanced techniques.

Applying Shisochin's Wisdom

Shisochin begins in Sanchin dachi, a stance that promotes a sense of rootedness, encourages controlled breathing, and enhances awareness of the centerline. From this strong foundation, the form transitions into Ayumi dachi, or the walking stance, which emphasizes forward movement while maintaining a connection to the ground. This progression continues into Zenkutsu dachi, the front stance, where practitioners focus on generating momentum and projection. The movement evolves further into Kosa dachi, the cross-legged stance, along with various transitional postures that highlight the importance of angular redirection and close-body control, weaving together a fluid expression of power and precision.

This blend of movement teaches adaptability: low when stability is required, high when fluidity is necessary. The movements are short and efficient, almost economical in nature, reflecting the kata's emphasis on real-world application.

In practicing Shisochin, key techniques and their applications, or bunkai, are vital for understanding the art's depth. The focus primarily rests on kaisho waza, or open-hand techniques, which prevail over the limited use of closed-fist strikes. Techniques such as palm-heel strikes, spear hands, and finger jabs underscore the importance of both precision and control, enabling practitioners to effectively target vulnerable areas such as joints, the neck, or specific pressure points.

Another significant aspect of Shisochin is the concept of muchimi, or heavy, sticky body movement. This principle emphasizes that even movements that appear light possess substantial weight and intent, which contributes to the overall effectiveness of each technique.

Vital-point strikes, the principles of projections, and tuite are all crucial as they are intricately woven into the transitions, often concealed within the flowing motions of practice. For example, practitioners may initiate hooks to an opponent's limb and seamlessly follow these with sweeps, or combine blocks with pulls in a fluid manner.

Central to the philosophy of Shisochin is the concept of simultaneous countering. Unlike many later Japanese karate styles, this system rarely involves isolated "blocks." Instead, it teaches practitioners to defend and attack in a single, unified motion, which is a distinctive characteristic of Okinawan karate. The internal rhythm shifts between whipping explosiveness and tensile coiling. One moment is rooted; the next moment is released; embodying the Goju principle of hard and soft.

Shisochin's Diverse Paths

Shisochin is one of the core kata in Goju-ryu karate, practiced widely across Okinawa and in affiliated lineages around the world. However, there are small yet significant variations among different schools.

In practicing Shisochin, various schools adopt different breathing techniques. Some emphasize a strong, audible ibuki breathing style rooted in the Sanchin tradition, while others prioritize a more relaxed and natural rhythm. Additionally, the mechanics of palm strikes, specifically the shōtei strikes, vary across lineages in terms of height, angle, and the way they are chambered. The stepping patterns also differ; some versions may open to various quadrants, reflecting the individual focus of different instructors.

Outside of Goju-ryu, Shisochin's influence is more limited, but its strategic philosophy has made its way into other martial arts systems, particularly those that emphasize grappling or close-quarters interception. The theorized historical connection to Sochin suggests that its movements may share a common lineage with other kata that have been adapted or renamed over time.

Some practitioners propose that the kata was originally designed for urban self-defense, suitable for narrow streets, close proximity, and chaotic environments, making it relevant for modern combatives training.

Shisochin's Lasting Impact

Shisochin is not a flamboyant kata. It may not be the most athletic, the most spectacular, or the most widely taught form, but within its understated structure lies a concentrated expression of Okinawan martial wisdom. It captures the moment where breath meets impact, where redirection becomes power, and where softness is not a sign of submission but a form of subtle dominance.

This kata reflects the maturity of a martial arts system; not just in a physical sense, but also philosophically. To fight in all directions is to live in all directions, to be aware, adaptable, and unshakably centered.

As Goju-ryu continues to evolve, Shisochin remains a kata of choice for serious practitioners; not because it's easy to master, but because true mastery reveals itself slowly, one palm strike at a time.

SANSERU
OKINAWA'S 36 TACTICS

Introduction to Sanseru

Sanseru does not respond to aggression with aggression. Instead, it avoids incoming attacks, redirects force, and counters with swift, targeted strikes. While other kata may focus on charging forward or holding their ground, Sanseru teaches a different lesson: the importance of survival and victory through outmaneuvering rather than overpowering.

As a mid-level kata in the Goju-ryu and Uechi-ryu systems, Sanseru, which literally means "Thirty-Six Hands" (三十六手), serves as a crucial connection between earlier conditioning forms like Sanchin and more advanced kata such as Suparinpei. With origins in Southern Chinese martial arts, specifically in styles like White Crane and Tiger Boxing, Sanseru emphasizes evasive footwork, joint manipulation, and focused striking.

This chapter will explore the strategic brilliance of Sanseru. We will examine how its evasive structure, development of internal power, and intriguing numerological name reflect deeper layers of combative and philosophical wisdom. Additionally, we will trace its journey from Chinese roots to its codification in Okinawa, investigate its various stylistic interpretations, and decode its ongoing significance as a marker of both technical and mental maturity.

Exploring Sanseru's Essence

- **Traditional Notation:** 三十六 (Sanseirū / Sanseru).
- **Script Breakdown:**
    - 三 "three";
    - 十 "ten";
    - 六 "six"
- **Core Meaning:** "Thirty-six [steps/hands]."
- **Modern Interpretations:** Numerological reading common (six times six energies, etc.).
- **Conflicting Ideas & Origins:** Number symbolism vs. concrete technique counts is debated.

The name "Sanseru," which translates to "Thirty-Six Hands" (三十六手), carries significant linguistic and historical meaning that has led to various interpretations. One common theory relates to numerical symbolism, suggesting that the number 36 is the product of 6 multiplied by 6. This symbolism is thought to represent the connection between the six senses, sight, sound, smell, taste, touch, and thought, and their interaction with six internal emotional states: joy, anger, love, hate, desire, and fear.

Another interpretation links "Thirty-Six" to 36 vital or forbidden points identified in traditional Chinese medicine and martial arts striking techniques, highlighting their importance in both health and combat practices. Some sources trace this concept back to the Ming Dynasty, where Feng Yiquan, a figure associated with the Ming military and Southern Chinese boxing, developed a system emphasizing 36 essential movements or strikes crucial for martial effectiveness. An intriguing theory from Okinawa suggests that "Thirty-Six" may refer to the 36 Chinese families who settled in Kume Village during the 14th century. Although this notion may hold symbolic rather than purely historical significance, it illustrates the deep cultural exchanges that shaped the martial traditions of the region.

Whether viewed from a numerical, spiritual, or anatomical perspective, the name "Sanseru" signifies depth, precision, and mastery. Unlike kata with poetic names, Sanseru's name suggests a repository of knowledge; measured technique rather than mythical narrative. It positions the kata as a deliberate and comprehensive system of principles, awaiting careful study by practitioners.

Sanseru's Historical Origins

The historical journey of Sanseru into Okinawan Karate begins with Kanryo Higaonna, who is widely credited with bringing the kata from Fuzhou, China. During his time in Fuzhou, he studied under various Chinese masters, including Ru Ru Ko. Sanseru likely entered Okinawan martial culture in the late 19th century, a period when Higaonna and others began importing forms that would later be systematized into the Naha-te tradition.

Higaonna's most prominent student, Chojun Miyagi, learned Sanseru directly from him and later formalized its place within his early 20th-century Goju-ryu curriculum. Miyagi may have played a significant role in refining or codifying the kata's structure, however, the fact that Kyoda Juhatsu, another student of Higaonna, also included Sanseru in his To'on-ryu system indicates that the kata was part of Higaonna's original teachings and predates Miyagi's formal contributions.

Applying Sanseru's Wisdom

The kata Sanseru serves as an important link between the internal conditioning of Sanchin and the more complex applications found in Suparinpei. Designed for close-range self-defense, it incorporates techniques such as joint locks, evasion, and pressure-point striking. Drawing inspiration from various Southern Chinese animal systems, including White Crane, Tiger, and possibly Dog boxing styles, the early sequence of the kata, particularly its stance and rhythm, bears a strong resemblance to Sanchin, reflecting a shared lineage. Meanwhile, its internal mechanics and conceptual connections with Suparinpei highlight its place within the numerically themed kata family.

To establish a solid foundation, Sanseru relies on various stances and movement principles. The Sanchin Dachi is used in the opening sequence to anchor the practitioner and harness their breath, while the Shiko Dachi and Neko Ashi Dachi enhance rotational power and maintain balance. Stepping and rotation techniques are essential for shifting angles, breaking an opponent's alignment, and gaining a tactical advantage. Core compression and expansion are vital for generating short-range power and fostering internal connectivity, which enhances the effectiveness of each technique.

Among Sanseru's key techniques and applications, the Morote Koken Waza, a double wrist movement at the end of the kata, stands out for its versatility; it can serve as a strike, throw, deflection, or method of arm control. The Kansetsu Geri, a side kick aimed at the opponent's knee joint, is designed to destabilize or incapacitate an opponent, while low front kicks target vulnerable areas such as the groin, thigh, or abdomen. Many movements typically considered blocks also function as strikes or structural collapses when applied with tactical intent.

Internally, Sanseru emphasizes rhythmic breathing, internal tension, and dynamic transitions. Concepts such as kime and kiai highlight timed bursts of power, focused through breath and hip compression. While chi development is a component for fostering internal energy, it is less emphasized than in Sanchin. Instead, the kata's breath-powered expansion, characterized by rhythmic breathing that closely ties with movement and tension cycling, plays a critical role in enhancing overall performance. This approach is designed to allow practitioners to refine their control over both movement and emotion under pressure.

Sanseru's Diverse Paths

The transmission history of Sanseru traces its evolution through several prominent Okinawan karate styles, each influenced by its unique lineage. The story begins with Higaonna Kanryo, who significantly impacted both Miyagi Chojun and Kyoda Juhatsu. This influence led to a branch in the lineage, resulting in Miyagi developing Goju-ryu and Kyoda founding To'on-ryu. Another major lineage traces its origins to Uechi Kanbun, who brought his Southern Chinese-influenced training to Okinawa, which ultimately led to the formation of Uechi-ryu. While all three styles share an ancestral link to Chinese martial arts, their interpretations of Sanseru reflect notable differences in practice.

These major stylistic variations are particularly significant. Goju-ryu is recognized for its complex transitions, dynamic pacing, and a distinctive double wrist technique. In contrast, To'on-ryu takes a different approach by excluding certain kicking techniques, such as mae geri and kansetsu geri, which are commonly found in Goju-ryu. Uechi-ryu emphasizes a unique structure and tempo, drawing inspiration from crane and tiger concepts, which sets it apart from the others.

The reasons for these variations are multifaceted. Okinawan teachers often tailored techniques for practical application, adapting them to better suit real life defensive scenarios and the specific needs of their students. This adaptation contributed to the divergence of lineages, as different instructors prioritized various principles, such as power versus flow and tension versus looseness. Additionally, ongoing refinement of the curriculum led to the restructuring and streamlining of kata for educational purposes, military training, and the demands of school systems.

The impact of these stylistic variations extends to other forms as well. The kata Suparinpei appears to build on the principles of Sanseru, while the techniques seen in Seipai share tactical elements, particularly in their use of folding strikes and low-line attacks. Furthermore, some contemporary bunkai systems have adopted Sanseru as a foundational model for pressure-point mapping and tuite flow.

Further enriching the narrative of Sanseru is the way its viewed; in many Goju-ryu dojos, the kata is regarded as the "gateway kata," serving as a significant milestone for students aspiring to achieve advanced black belt levels of bunkai. Additionally, several old Okinawan teachers have referred to Sanseru as the "strategy kata," highlighting its mental demands and the strategic thinking it requires, often placing greater emphasis on mental acuity than on physical exertion.

Sanseru's Lasting Impact

Sanseru represents a significant shift in strategy and mindset, guiding practitioners away from the idea of meeting force with force. Instead, it emphasizes absorbing, redirecting, and outmaneuvering an opponent. This approach encourages individuals to be measured, aware, and precise; qualities that are often more effective than brute strength in close combat. With its deep roots in Chinese martial arts and refined layers from Okinawa, Sanseru is one of the most intellectually and tactically rich katas in the Goju-ryu system.

Sanseru serves as both a technical connection and a philosophical landmark in Okinawan karate. Its teachings on evasion, economy of motion, and mental clarity extend well beyond the dojo. In a world frequently focused on speed and strength, Sanseru reminds us that subtlety, structure, and strategy are essential for winning real fights.

Section III - Advanced Kata

Consolidation, Depth, and Martial Compression

Advanced kata are more than just long sequences or collections of challenging techniques. Their true challenge lies in the depth of principles they embody and the level of integration they require from the practitioner. These are not kata meant to be memorized and performed; rather, they are to be deciphered.

In Okinawan karate, advanced kata often represent culmination forms. Kata like Gojushiho and Suparinpei compile earlier principles, incorporating them into new sequences and reconfiguring foundational concepts into multidirectional flow. Practitioners must master power, structure, and timing that shift seamlessly. The opponent is no longer viewed as a single attacker; instead, they represent a changing situation, which requires adaptability rather than mere execution.

Some advanced kata also function as preservation vaults, containing fragments of older systems that might otherwise be lost. Others are modern syntheses designed to integrate principles from various influences, be it Chinese, Okinawan, or Japanese, and present them as a cohesive whole. In both cases, the kata should be interpreted like a manuscript: not everything is literal, and some elements were intended for those who understand what lies beneath the surface.

Internal cultivation plays a more prominent role here, not in an esoteric sense, but as a necessary refinement. Timing alone is insufficient; movement must be continuous. Power must be generated without telegraphing intentions. Breathing should maintain a rhythm that enhances structure rather than disrupts it. Suparinpei, in particular, exemplifies this paradox: it is slow yet explosive, hard yet yielding, and direct yet circuitous; all at once.

These kata are not considered advanced because they are unattainable; rather, they require the student to become a different kind of practitioner in order to fully grasp their meaning.

SUPARINPEI
OKINAWA'S 108 STEPS

Introduction to Suparinpei

Among the kata of Okinawan Karate, Suparinpei is renowned for its scope, complexity, and symbolic significance. Often regarded as a culmination of previous forms, it represents a profound spiritual confrontation with the self.

Translating to "One Hundred and Eight Hands," Suparinpei is the longest and most technically demanding kata in the Goju-ryu system. While it is practiced in various Okinawan and Japanese styles today, its core structure can be traced back to Southern Chinese Kempo and Buddhist numerology. As the capstone kata of Goju-ryu, it integrates both internal and external principles, combining elements from earlier forms such as Sanchin, Sanseiryu, Seisan, and others into a comprehensive blueprint for martial and personal mastery.

This chapter will explore Suparinpei's historical roots, technical depth, symbolic meaning, and its evolution across multiple lineages. We will argue that this kata serves not only as an advanced form but also as a compendium of combat principles layered with philosophical significance; a living record of how Okinawan karate evolved under Chinese influence and a Buddhist worldview.

Exploring Suparinpei's Essence

- **Traditional Notation:** 壱百零八 / 百八 (Suparinpei/Hyakuhachi).
- **Script Breakdown:**
  - 壱 "one";
  - 百 "hundred";
  - 零 "zero";
  - 八 "eight"
- **Core Meaning:** "One hundred eight [hands]."
- **Modern Interpretations:** Linked to Buddhist numerology/Fujian boxing sets.
- **Conflicting Ideas & Origins:** Whether 108 denotes techniques or spiritual numerology varies among lines.

The name Suparinpei (壱百零八), often translated as "One Hundred and Eight Hands," holds profound symbolic significance. It is composed of Japanese characters: 壱 (Ichi), meaning "one"; 百 (Hyaku), meaning "one hundred"; 零 (Rei), meaning "zero"; and 八 (Hachi), meaning "eight." Together, these characters read as "108." This method of writing the number is unusual in contemporary Japanese, typically reserved for specific contexts like phone numbers or numerology. However, it was a common practice in 18th-century China, further linking the kata to its deep Chinese roots. The numerical value of 108 is central to the kata's identity and is associated with an earlier name, "Pechurin," which may imply "108 steps in succession," suggesting a sense of progression and immense complexity.

The number 108 carries significant meaning in Buddhism, Taoism, and Chinese martial traditions. In Buddhism, it represents the total number of worldly defilements or desires that a person must overcome on the path to enlightenment. This journey transcends numerical value—it's an endeavor toward spiritual clarity and liberation from attachments. Additionally, 108 can be viewed as a culmination of intricate mathematical and philosophical principles: the six senses (sight, sound, smell, taste, touch, and thought) multiplied by three qualities (good, bad, and neutral), combined with two origins of experience (internal and external), and expanded across three dimensions of time (past, present, and future).

This numerology goes beyond mere calculation, weaving a rich tapestry of meaning that suggests a holistic and spiritual confrontation. Every New Year's Eve in Japan, Buddhist temples ring their bells 108 times, with each chime signifying the purification of one defilement. Naming a kata after this number indicates not only martial completeness but also a spiritual challenge. Thus, Suparinpei serves both as a collection of combat principles and as a metaphor for transcendence.

Suparinpei's Historical Origins

Historically, Suparinpei was influenced by Southern Chinese Kempo, particularly the styles of White Crane, Dragon, and Tiger. There is also a notable, though often mythical, connection to Yue Shi San Shou, or "Yue Fei's 108 Hands." This kata is believed to be a synthesis of earlier Pechurin forms, of which only the highest level has been preserved in the Okinawan transmission.

Suparinpei, as we recognize it today, began its journey from Fuzhou, China, to Okinawa during the late 19th century. Kanryo Higaonna is widely credited with introducing the kata, having learned it during his training under Ryu Ryu Ko.

The creation and codification of this kata aimed to preserve advanced combat principles, including methods for harnessing internal energy, controlling limbs, and striking through acupressure techniques. Furthermore, Suparinpei reflects deeper spiritual and philosophical themes through its martial movements. This indicates a deliberate effort to create a comprehensive final form, integrating elements from earlier Goju-ryu kata such as Sanchin, Seisan, Sanseru, and Seipai, and weaving them into a single expansive blueprint for both martial and personal mastery.

Applying Suparinpei's Wisdom

Suparinpei is a masterclass in structural integrity and power redirection, requiring a sophisticated understanding of stances and movement principles. The kata features various stances, including Sanchin Dachi, Shiko Dachi, and Neko Ashi Dachi, each providing a different structural base for effectively shifting momentum. Its movements showcase a dynamic rhythm, transitioning between tight spirals and sharp linear bursts that reflect the shift from soft deflections to hard counters.

This fluidity is enhanced through rotational mechanics, where the hips and shoulders pivot at various angles, adding power and the ability to disrupt an opponent's structure.

The kata's extensive repertoire of techniques is heavily inspired by the movements of cranes, incorporating whipping wrist strikes, hooking hands, and evasive angles designed to maintain fluid motion. Practitioners apply tuite principles, utilizing joint locks and pressure points to incapacitate their opponents. Strategies involving multiple grabs, releases, and holds are employed to unbalance or disable adversaries before delivering a decisive strike; double-handed applications to control an opponent's arms and target their centerline emphasize its focus on complex, close-range engagement.

On an internal level, Suparinpei integrates breath control with its tempo shifts, enabling both explosive power and sustained delivery. Achieving kime (focused power) and zanshin (heightened awareness) necessitates extreme precision and emotional discipline. The kata promotes the cultivation of ki or chi as a means of aligning the body and spirit through sustained, mindful practice. From a pedagogical perspective, Suparinpei serves as a synthesis of skills, reinforcing concepts from earlier forms such as Seisan, Sanseru, and Sanchin. The repetitive nature of its techniques and the use of application drills allow practitioners to break down the kata into shorter segments, isolating and mastering key principles for both martial and personal growth.

Suparinpei's Diverse Paths

The transmission and evolution of Suparinpei across different styles demonstrate its lasting impact and technical versatility. Following in Higaonna's footsteps, his senior student and the founder of Goju-ryu, Chojun Miyagi, played a crucial role in preserving this kata, codifying it as a pinnacle form within his curriculum. Another of Higaonna's students, Kenwa Mabuni, also incorporated Suparinpei into the Shito ryu curriculum, ensuring its preservation across various lineages. The kata's influence extended into later generations, with Masutatsu Oyama introducing a version into the Kyokushin style through Nei-Chu So, and more recently, Hakoishi Katsumi reconstructed it for Wado-ryu, which showcases its enduring complexity and significance.

The practice of Suparinpei varies considerably across these styles. The version most widely practiced today is found in Goju-ryu, known for its length, complex tempo, and embodiment of the style's core principles. In contrast, Shito-ryu often presents a more linear delivery and a clearer breakdown of applications, reflecting Mabuni's methodical approach. The Wado-ryu adaptation, reconstructed by Hakoishi Katsumi, aligns the kata with Wado's foundational principles, offering a modern interpretation. In Kyokushin, while Suparinpei is occasionally featured in high-level demonstrations, it is often presented in a simplified form.

These variations can be attributed to several factors. The kata's extensive length often leads instructors to simplify it for teaching purposes. Different ryu philosophies also influence its interpretation, emphasizing principles such as flow versus explosion or hardness versus softness. Historically, some versions may have been lost or preserved only in part, necessitating reconstruction and adaptation over time.

Suparinpei serves as a crucial index kata, encompassing techniques and transitions from earlier forms like Sanchin, Seisan, and Sanseru. Many practitioners view it as a "collection kata" or a compendium of the system's most advanced principles. This role is reinforced by the legends and anecdotes surrounding the kata. Some practitioners report experiencing spiritual or emotional breakthroughs during training, owing to its intensity and profound depth. In certain dojos, it is said that Suparinpei was once reserved exclusively for senior instructors, highlighting its revered status within the martial arts community as the final technical and philosophical challenge.

Suparinpei's Lasting Impact

Suparinpei represents not just an endpoint but a distillation of Goju-ryu. As the most advanced kata in the system, it synthesizes a wide range of techniques, stances, and tactics, while also reflecting a worldview centered on self-refinement, confronting one's ego, and achieving mastery through repetition. It serves not only as a record of combative principles but also as a blueprint for inner development.

In an era when many kata are practiced primarily for aesthetics or competition, Suparinpei resists simplification. Its layered structure, spiritual numerology, and profound depth in combat defy casual performance. For serious students, it remains a technical Rosetta Stone and a spiritual test; a form that challenges not just the body, but the whole person.

SEIPAI

OKINAWA'S 18 DEFENSES

Introduction to Seipai

Few kata inspire as much symbolic speculation as Seipai. Its name, typically translated as "Eighteen Hands," raises an intriguing question: What does "eighteen" signify? Is it a code for combative strategy, a nod to numerology, or a reference to pressure point theory? This very ambiguity is central to the kata's identity, while its movements themselves demand careful study.

Seipai is a revered and advanced form within the Naha-te tradition, distinguished by its unique rhythm, which blends hard and soft power, stillness and sudden movement. Deeply rooted in Southern Chinese martial arts, particularly Fujian White Crane, the kata was systematized in Okinawa by Kanryo Higaonna and later passed down through Chojun Miyagi's Goju-ryu system. It is characterized by the use of circular motions, body evasion, joint manipulations, and a profound internal logic shaped by the yin-yang duality of hard and soft.

In the following sections, we will view Seipai not as a static relic but as a living cipher. We will explore the multiple meanings of "eighteen," trace the kata's lineage and transformation, and analyze its complex techniques. Through this exploration, we will see how Seipai has been both partially preserved and partially obscured by the evolution of Okinawan karate.

Exploring Seipai's Essence

- **Traditional Notation:** 十八 (Seipai).
- **Script Breakdown:**

    o 十 "ten";

    o 八 "eight"

- **Core Meaning:** "Eighteen."
- **Modern Interpretations:** Often taken as a numeric set from southern Chinese curricula.
- **Conflicting Ideas & Origins:** As with number-kata, intent of numerals differs by tradition.

The name Seipai (十八手) is derived from Kanji characters that literally translate to "Eighteen Hands." The first character, 十 (ju), represents the number ten; the second character, 八 (hachi), signifies eight; and the final character, 手 (te), translates to "hands." While this numerical description seems straightforward, it conceals a wealth of deeper symbolic and practical meanings.

The pronunciation "Seipai" comes from the Fujian dialect, where "Sei" means ten and "Pai" means eight. This connection strongly links the kata to its Chinese heritage and aligns it with Southern Shaolin numerological naming conventions (for example, Sanseru = 36, Suparinpei = 108).

The number 18 has inspired various interpretations within the martial arts community. Literally, it may represent a specific set of 18 techniques or combat applications. On a more symbolic and philosophical level, the number is rooted in Buddhist cosmology, emerging from the multiplication of the six senses by the three states of experience: good, bad, and neutral. Additionally, some interpret it as an encoded reference to a striking system targeting vital pressure points, particularly suggesting that it represents half of Sanseru's total of 36 vital targets. A more poetic interpretation suggests that the number refers to "18 guards for the King," implying an elite approach to protective strategies.

In East Asian numerology and Buddhist philosophy, the number 18 is significant; it represents completeness through the balance of dualistic elements. If Sanseru's 36 is seen as a more complex combative framework, Seipai's 18 may symbolize a distilled or complementary system. In this sense, the name positions the kata as both a tactical tool and a philosophical invitation, encouraging practitioners to explore its movements for both practical application and deeper meaning.

Seipai's Historical Origins

An advanced kata in the Naha-te tradition, Seipai represents a significant blend of Chinese and Okinawan martial arts. Its historical development is strongly influenced by two key figures. The transmission of Seipai began with Kanryo Higaonna, an essential master who studied Southern Chinese Kempo during his multiple visits to Fujian Province, China. His training under masters such as Ru Ro Ko (possibly Xie Zhongxiang) laid the groundwork for the Naha-te tradition. Seipai likely entered Okinawan practice when Higaonna returned from China in the late 19th century, a time when Chinese influence was prominent in port cities like Naha, just before karate began to undergo widespread Japanization.

Higaonna likely selected or synthesized Seipai for its strategic balance of close-quarter grappling, body conditioning, and evasive movement. The kata's internal logic and complexity made it an ideal means for teaching principles of softness within hard techniques, making it suitable for advanced students. His foremost student, Chojun Miyagi, later incorporated Seipai into his Goju-ryu curriculum, further emphasizing the contrast between hard and soft techniques and focusing on internal development.

From the Goju-ryu tradition, Seipai's influence spread to other lineages, notably entering Kyokushin under Mas Oyama, who learned it from Nei-Chu So, a student of Gogen Yamaguchi.

Seipai clearly exhibits influences from Southern Chinese martial systems, particularly White Crane and Tiger Boxing. While no definitive Chinese ancestor has been identified, the kata's body mechanics, rhythm, and close-range focus suggest a direct link to Southern Shaolin temple forms. It is widely believed that Seipai shares ancestral characteristics with other Naha-te katas like Sanseru and Suparinpei, reinforcing its position within a family of martial arts rooted in the martial philosophies of southern China.

Applying Seipai's Wisdom

The kata Seipai is a challenging study in foundational stances, evasive movement, and the smooth transition between hard and soft techniques. It is characterized by rooted postures that emphasize stability and the development of internal energy. Movement within Seipai is determined by body evasion, employing angular entries and exits to avoid an opponent's attacks. This fluid, flowing footwork often contrasts with sudden, snapping techniques, embodying the core Goju-ryu duality of hard and soft.

Seipai's technical repertoire serves as a masterclass in close-range tactics and sophisticated bunkai. Its movements subtly incorporate joint locks and tuite, including elbow manipulations, wrist controls, and takedowns. Some interpretations highlight precise strikes to vital pressure points in the neck, ribs, and inner thigh. The kata also features circular off-balancing motions that suggest short-range grappling and throwing techniques. By training a practitioner's defensive and offensive actions in all four cardinal directions, Seipai fosters a deep awareness of the surrounding space, enabling seamless adaptation between tight infighting and longer-range strikes.

Ultimately, successful performance of Seipai requires not only technical precision but also the integration of timed breathing, kime, and zanshin (lingering awareness) as essential components of the form.

Seipai's Diverse Paths

Primarily passed down from Kanryo Higaonna to his top student, Chojun Miyagi, Seipai has been preserved with remarkable integrity. Today, Goju-ryu schools are the main custodians of this kata, maintaining the classic hard-soft dynamics that are essential to its practice. From this foundational lineage, Seipai has spread into various derivative systems, each adapting the form to reflect its unique philosophy. For instance, Shito-ryu introduces slight variations in tempo and footwork, adding a distinctive flair to its movements, while Kyokushin, which adopted the form through Nei-Chu So, often emphasizes raw power at the expense of the internal nuances prioritized by other styles. Each of these variations contributes to the rich tapestry of karate, showcasing the diverse philosophies and teaching methods across different schools.

The reasons for these variations are multifaceted. Different lineages interpret the concept of bunkai (application) in unique ways, leading to diverse understandings and applications of the kata. Additionally, the teaching needs in contemporary settings have shifted the focus toward showcasing visible power, particularly in competitive contexts, which often emphasizes sport over traditional practices. Lastly, personal adaptations by senior masters have significantly influenced how the kata has evolved within their respective systems.

Seipai's structural template, characterized by seamless transitions between hardness and fluidity, has profoundly impacted the later composition and interpretation of other Goju-ryu katas. It serves as a crucial midpoint in the curriculum, bridging the foundational Sanchin and the expansive Suparinpei. Anecdotal evidence further enriches its legacy, suggesting that Higaonna used Seipai to assess his students' ability to maintain structure under pressure. One popular, though speculative, tale claims that the kata was a training tool for defending dignitaries, reflecting the poetic idea of "18 guards for the King." This legend underscores the kata's perceived sophistication and elite status within the Goju-ryu curriculum.

Seipai's Lasting Impact

Seipai represents a fusion of Southern Chinese strategy and Okinawan pragmatism. It is a kata characterized by contrasts, skillfully integrating tempo, range, force, and intention. The number "eighteen" in its name may refer to a specific number of techniques, core principles, or deep spiritual concepts. Regardless, the kata itself presents a rich and comprehensive curriculum.

Today, Seipai stands as a cornerstone of Goju-ryu karate and serves as a timeless example of how kata can convey layered knowledge across generations. Its combination of symbolic depth and practical application ensures its ongoing significance in both traditional practice and modern combat exploration.

JION

OKINAWA'S TEMPLE STRENGTH

Introduction to Jion

There is a deceptive stillness in the opening salutation of Jion, quietly reminiscent of prayer or perhaps a vow. Many observers see this posture and assume it to be a ceremonial flourish, a remnant of some imagined Shaolin theater. However, behind that gesture lies a depth of history and intent that cannot be easily overlooked. Jion is a kata that is both revered and shrouded in ambiguity; its simplicity concealing sophisticated fundamentals, and its purpose debated even among seasoned karate practitioners.

This chapter will trace the layered history of Jion, dissect the meaning behind its name, investigate its contested origins, and explore its defining technical characteristics and variations. In doing so, it will position Jion not only as a kata of foundational importance but as a lens through which to examine the cultural and technical crosscurrents that shaped modern Okinawan and Japanese karate.

Exploring Jion's Essence

- **Traditional Notation:** 慈恩 (Jion).
- **Script Breakdown:**
  - 慈 "benevolence";
  - 恩 "grace/favor."
- **Core Meaning:** "Compassion and benevolence," or a reference to "Jion-ji" temple.
- **Modern Interpretations:** Shotokan literature ties title to Buddhist overtones or temple associations.
- **Conflicting Ideas & Origins:** Whether it stems from a temple name or a teacher's sobriquet remains debated.

The prevailing evidence indicates that the name "Jion" was originally, and indeed our earliest confirmed recording, ere written using the Kanji characters 慈恩. This is supported by a theory mentioned in Funakoshi's second edition of "Karate-Do Kyohan" (1973), which suggests that this name or its characters appear frequently in Chinese literature and may be linked to a Buddhist temple or saint named Jion.

The characters for Jion, 慈恩, are often translated as "mercy and grace" or "compassion and gratitude." A more literal interpretation would be "Mercy (慈) + Kindness/Benevolence (恩)." However, many Shotokan-based sources, such as Shotokan Karate Online, translate it as "Temple Sound," possibly referencing a different kanji homonym (寺音).

Unlike many other kata, which have been renamed from Okinawan to Japanese pronunciations or assigned entirely new names, Jion has largely retained its original Okinawan name. This continuity suggests a deep-rooted historical association with its Kanji characters.

The kata may be named after Jion-ji, a Chinese Buddhist temple purported to have housed martial monks. Alternatively, its name might reflect a moral ideal: compassion through power, or restraint through strength. Regardless of its semantic origin, the name suggests a kata that embodies both martial and philosophical elements.

Jion is often grouped with Jiin and Jitte, two similarly structured forms. All three begin with the same distinctive salutation, sometimes referred to as "Jiai no Kamae," which many researchers associate with a traditional Chinese greeting common in Ming-era martial arts. Whether symbolizing humility, readiness, or fraternity, this gesture connects the "temple kata" into a thematic family.

Jion's Historical Origins

The exact creator of Jion remains unknown. However, it is frequently attributed to the lineage of Sokon Matsumura, who may have acquired or adapted it during his documented travels to Fujian, China. Some theories propose that Matsumura encountered a proto-version of Jion at a Buddhist temple known as Jion-ji, incorporating it into his Tomari-based practice. Later, Anko Itosu is credited with refining and systematizing the form for inclusion into public school karate curricula in the early 20th century.

If Matsumura indeed introduced Jion to Okinawa, its origins would date to the mid-19th century, roughly concurrent with his return from service in Satsuma and his consolidation of Okinawan fighting methods. However, its wide dissemination came later, through Itosu's reforms around the Meiji era (late 1800s to early 1900s), when kata like Jion were codified for pedagogical use in the Okinawan school system.

Jion's simplicity and structural clarity made it an ideal candidate for both instructional and evaluative use. It offered a platform to test a student's ability to perform basic techniques with power, stability, and precision, without relying on the flashier elements of higher forms. The kata's advancing block-counter sequences reflect battlefield pragmatism, while its symmetrical layout lends itself to group instruction.

The presumed Chinese influence is difficult to dismiss. The hypothesis that Jion derived from Jion-ji, a Chinese temple with martial connections, is repeated in Japanese texts—especially by Shotokan patriarchs like Hirokazu Kanazawa. Nevertheless, Okinawan sources are less certain. Scholars like Yannick Sensei, who have examined pre-war literature and oral history, point out the kata's absence in many older Okinawan curricula. This raises the possibility that Jion, or at least its modern form, may be a Japanese-era consolidation or adaptation of an earlier Tomari-based form.

Applying Jion's Wisdom

The kata Jion is a demanding study in clarity of structure and foundational power generation. Its heavy reliance on Kiba Dachi (horse stance) and Zenkutsu Dachi (front stance) challenges the practitioner to maintain unwavering stability while simultaneously generating explosive power. In some Shito-ryu interpretations, Kokutsu Dachi (back stance) also appears more frequently, introducing valuable variations in weight distribution and transitional flow.

Critical to Jion's essence are the seamless transitions between the square and angled body positions. These shifts are not merely stylistic; they are foundational to understanding the timing and biomechanics necessary for direct engagement and evasive angling in combat.

The hallmark of Jion is its forward-driving rhythm of block, counter, advance. Its movements are deliberately unflashy, devoid of spinning kicks or acrobatics. Instead, the kata emphasizes crisp, committed basics: downward blocks, middle punches, reinforced strikes, and controlled shifts of stance. Every technique in Jion invites multiple interpretations. For instance, a rising block might subtly double as a chin strike, or a downward block could conceal a joint break or takedown.

The applications of Jion's techniques are profoundly practical. They include grabbing and throwing initiated directly from the initial kamae position, as well as effective parrying and entering against punches. Practitioners learn to disrupt an opponent's balance through low strikes while advancing, and the kata seamlessly incorporates chokes and joint manipulations embedded within what may appear to be simple motions. Jion's true strength lies in the clarity it offers; every technique is laid bare, highlighting any flaws in the practitioner's mechanics and compelling them to refine their fundamental movements to an exceptional level.

Jion's Diverse Paths

Jion's path from Okinawa to Japan followed the same general route as many forms standardized by Itosu and later taught by Funakoshi Gichin. In Japan, Jion gained prominence in Shotokan and subsequently spread through Shito-ryu and Wado-ryu lineages.

There are several major stylistic variations among different karate styles. Shotokan is characterized by its linear and powerful techniques, placing a strong emphasis on deep stances and large, expansive movements. In contrast, Shito-ryu adopts a more circular approach, often incorporating alternate stances and nuanced footwork that adds a level of complexity to its practice. Meanwhile, Wado-ryu incorporates softer transitions, a reflection of its jujutsu influence, which gives it a unique fluidity compared to other styles. Additionally, Kyudokan stands out with notable differences from traditional Japanese interpretations, retaining a distinctly Okinawan flavor in its techniques and approach.

Focusing on specific interpretations, Hanashiro Chomo's version of Jion is still practiced in select Okinawan dojos, preserving a traditional lineage. On the other hand, Yabu Kentsu's interpretation has been preserved in To'on-ryu, located in Oita Prefecture, highlighting a pre-war transmission of karate knowledge and practice.

Connection to Ji'in and Jitte

These three kata have more in common than just their name prefix. Their structural and philosophical similarities, especially in the opening salutation, indicate either a shared origin or a deliberate grouping by later instructors. Whether these kata were derived from a temple-based system or linked retrospectively by educators like Itosu remains an open question.

Jion's Lasting Impact

Jion is often misunderstood as merely a "beginner's advanced kata;" something taught for show or rank. But under that veneer lies a form of quiet depth, technical rigor, and philosophical grace. Its lack of flair is precisely what makes it indispensable. Jion demands that one strip away the extraneous and examine the marrow of Karate: stance, timing, power, clarity.

Whether born in a Chinese temple, crafted in the halls of Tomari, or reassembled in the pedagogical forges of Meiji-era Okinawa, Jion endures. It speaks with the voice of tradition, not through spectacle, but through the echo of steady footsteps, unyielding stance, and the silent prayer of fist enclosed by open hand.

JITTE
OKINAWA'S TEN DEFENSES

Introduction to Jitte

Jitte occupies a unique and intriguing position within the canon of karate. Its name suggests a significant martial advantage, yet its structure implies qualities of restraint, evasion, and strategic positioning. Some believe it prepares practitioners to defend against armed attackers, while others argue that both its name and form reference the Edo-period police weapon of the same name. Jitte is both enigmatic and powerful, making it a kata that is often misunderstood.

As an advanced form linked to both the Shuri-te and Tomari-te traditions, Jitte is widely practiced today in styles such as Shotokan and Shito-ryu, although its precise origins remain unclear. It is particularly notable for its strong open-hand techniques, distinct stances, and its focus on defending against armed attackers, especially the bo. Thematic elements within Jitte also resonate with those found in the kata Jion and Ji'in, suggesting a shared heritage with Chinese martial arts or Buddhist temple systems.

This chapter will examine the symbolic ambiguity of Jitte, its complex technical content, and the varying theories regarding its origin and purpose. We will argue that Jitte is not simply a kata for weapon defense or merely a derivative of Chinese boxing; rather, it serves as a model of tactical composure, providing control, precision, and adaptability in situations that require more than just brute force.

Exploring Jitte's Essence

- **Traditional Notation:** 十手 (Jitte/Jutte).
- **Script Breakdown:**
    - 十 "ten";
    - 手 "hand";
    - also a police truncheon name.
- **Core Meaning:** "Ten hands" (metaphor for many defenses) or reference to the weapon.
- **Modern Interpretations:** Often taught alongside Jion/Jiin as a "temple" triad.
- **Conflicting Ideas & Origins:** Whether title refers to numerical metaphor or to the jutte weapon is unsettled.

The name "Jitte" (十手) is made up of the kanji characters for "ten" (十, Ju) and "hand" (手, Te), which translates literally to "Ten Hands." This translation raises interesting discussions about the kata's true meaning. One common interpretation suggests that the name implies a fighter's exceptional skill, enabling them to deal with multiple threats as if they had the power of ten hands. This may indicate techniques for disarming opponents or engaging several attackers at once.

Interestingly, "jitte" also refers to an actual weapon: an iron truncheon with a single prong used by police during Japan's Edo period. This weapon was designed for catching, controlling, or disarming swords and staves. The movements and techniques within the kata resemble the use of this weapon. Since the kanji characters for both the kata and the weapon are the same, there is speculation about whether the kata was named after the weapon or if its name arises from a purely metaphorical origin.

Regardless of its exact origin, the name "Jitte" conveys a sense of martial authority and mastery. Whether it refers to a weapon or symbolizes a fighter's ability to manage chaos, the name embodies the skill to confront multiple threats with confidence and precision. If the kata symbolizes "ten hands," it suggests a profound level of combative awareness and mastery over various attack vectors.

Jitte's Historical Origins

While the origins of Jitte are surrounded by mystery, as no single historical figure can be credited with its creation, its roots likely trace back to the 18th or early 19th century; a time before Okinawan karate was introduced into the public school system. Many theories connect Jitte to early Okinawan pioneers and the influence of Chinese martial arts. For instance, some scholars speculate that the kata may have originated with a Chinese martial monk who inspired figures like Kusanku, Sakugawa, and Matsumura, either directly or through the transmission of Chinese boxing techniques.

Later, Anko Itosu, a pivotal figure in modern karate development, may have played a crucial role in systematizing or preserving Jitte while synthesizing various forms for his school curricula. It was Gichin Funakoshi, after his training in the Shuri-te tradition, who formally integrated Jitte into the Shotokan curriculum. He valued its open-hand techniques and recognized its potential for weapon defense, emphasizing its practical applications in martial training.

The primary motivation behind the creation of Jitte seems to have been a response to armed threats, particularly against the bo staff. The kata's emphasis on open-hand techniques and control gestures suggests a focus on neutralizing and restraining an attacker rather than solely destroying them. Jitte was likely developed to complement harder, more linear martial arts forms, offering a counterpoint rooted in adaptability and the principles of soft-handed control.

In exploring its influences, similarities can be observed with Chinese Arhat Boxing, or Luohan Quan, as Jitte's opening posture and fluid footwork closely resemble certain Shaolin forms. Additionally, elements of White Crane Kung Fu may be reflected in its evasive footwork and redirection-based defense techniques. This has led to speculation that Jitte, along with other forms like Jion and Ji'in, may have originated from a monastic combat system, though this idea remains unproven.

Applying Jitte's Wisdom

The kata Jitte is built on a foundation of diverse stances and fluid movement principles. The Zenkutsu Dachi is used for powerful, linear attacks, while the Kiba Dachi provides a stable base for defending against threats from multiple directions, while in styles like Shito-ryu, the Kokutsu Dachi is particularly emphasized for its ability to facilitate quick redirection and defensive maneuvers. Throughout the kata, practitioners must maintain a high degree of 360° awareness, with frequent directional shifts highlighting the importance of being prepared for threats from all sides.

Central to Jitte's technical repertoire is the unique Tate Shuto, a vertical knife-hand technique that can serve as a strike, a redirection, or a setup for a lock. High blocks are often interpreted as defenses against the bo, underscoring the kata's focus on weapon defense, and the principles of hooking and sweeping suggest possibilities for joint manipulations, creating opportunities for off-balancing throws or grappling-like redirection. This emphasis on control reveals a deeper understanding of uke, the practitioner receiving the attack. Many movements in Jitte are not just blocks; they represent a seamless transition from a defensive maneuver into a control move, strike, or finishing technique. This adaptability is essential in close-range engagements where, despite the presence of large stances, many applications occur in tight quarters.

Having mentioned the modern interpretation of Jitte as a kata that encodes empty-hand defense against weapons, it's important to note Funakoshi's own perspective on this. According to Facebook posts, he stated in a 1914 article that Passai (Bassai) was the best kata for learning techniques against a bo attack, not Jitte. This suggests a potential misinterpretation or later adaptation of Jitte's bunkai.

On an internal level, Jitte is as much a mental practice as it is a physical one. Heijoshin, or maintaining a calm mind under duress, is a key principle for managing stress during combat. This is complemented by Muchimi, a heavy, sticky motion evident in control-based responses, emphasizing being grounded and fully aware of one's movements. Zanshin, or lingering awareness, is constantly reinforced through the kata's directional changes, keeping the practitioner mentally present and sharp. The relationship between breathing and kime (focused power) is also vital, as the rhythm of breath accentuates sudden changes in intensity and focus, allowing for quick adaptation and mental clarity in the midst of action. Together, these elements create a holistic approach to mental and physical discipline.

Jitte's Diverse Paths

The transmission history of Jitte reveals its journey through several prominent styles. Experts suggest that the kata's tactical elements of evasion and control may reflect influences from Tomari-te, and there is a speculative link to Fuzhou-based Chuan Fa that adds an intriguing layer to its origins.

These different lineages have led to significant stylistic variations. The Shotokan version of Jitte is characterized by its linear emphasis, long stances, and a straightforward approach to techniques. In contrast, Shito-ryu offers a more intricate style with complex hand transitions, diverse footwork, and a stronger focus on traditional bunkai. Wado-ryu, on the other hand, integrates elements from jujutsu, resulting in lighter body mechanics. Additionally, hybrid systems like Cuong Nhu and Suzucho Karate showcase unique applications by blending techniques from various influences.

The primary reasons for these divergences are philosophical and pedagogical. For example, Shotokan prioritizes strength and linearity, while Shito-ryu values complexity and strict adherence to tradition. These contrasting priorities have led to different interpretations of the same form. Over time, curriculums have been adjusted to integrate Jitte into broader kata progression systems. As with many forms, today's versions may only partially reflect their original intentions, as some elements have been lost or reinterpreted over the centuries.

Jitte's influence extends far beyond its own form. Its emphasis on open-hand control has influenced or parallels other kata that share similar themes, such as Jion, Ji'in, and Passai Dai. Furthermore, Jitte's multi-directional flow serves as a crucial precursor to the more complex spatial awareness explored in later black belt forms, highlighting how foundational kata can shape and inform advanced practices.

Jitte's Lasting Impact

Jitte is a kata filled with paradoxes. Although it is named after a weapon, it is practiced empty-handed. At first glance, it may seem simple, yet it is layered with tactical nuances. The kata implies the ability to fight multiple opponents, but it rewards practitioners who learn to neutralize attacks with control rather than overpowering them with force. Its techniques focus on strategic receiving, manipulation, and redirection, showcasing a sophisticated approach to combat.

Jitte has remained popular due to its versatility and symbolic significance. It continues to be practiced in Shotokan, Shito-ryu, Wado-ryu, and various hybrid systems. Whether seen as a template for weapon defense, a collection of open-hand control techniques, or a reflection of the Chinese roots of Okinawan martial arts, Jitte stands out as one of karate's most strategic and understated forms; a true test of composure and skill.

JI'IN

OKINAWA'S GENTLE POWER

Introduction to Ji'in

Among the many katas with names that evoke Buddhist themes and Chinese mystique, few are as puzzling as Ji'in. Removed from the Japan Karate Association (JKA) syllabus and often overshadowed by its more well-known counterpart, Jion, Ji'in remains a kata with an unresolved identity. It is a form rich in symbolism, sharp directional shifts, and layered meanings. Many practitioners encounter Ji'in only to forget it soon after, but beneath its compact structure lies something profound.

Like Jion and Jitte, Ji'in begins with the distinctive left-hand-over-right fist kamae, a salute said to reference Chinese martial etiquette or Buddhist origins. Ji'in sets itself apart with its intricate footwork, complex transitions, and demanding static techniques. Although it is considered a black belt-level kata in Shotokan and is practiced in several other systems, Ji'in is often relegated to the margins of curricula; known but not deeply studied. Its compact structure and enigmatic name continue to provoke curiosity, especially as its presence in modern syllabi has diminished.

This chapter will explore Ji'in's multifaceted character: its linguistic ambiguity, its potential connections to Chinese and Tomari-te systems, its compressed yet expressive structure, and its thematic relationships with Jion and Jitte. We will argue that Ji'in embodies a transitional kata whose strategic value lies in its dynamic control, psychological intent, and meditative composure.

Exploring Ji'in's Essence

- **Traditional Notation:** 慈陰 (Ji'in).
- **Script Breakdown:**
    - 慈 "compassion";
    - 陰 "shade/hidden."
- **Core Meaning:** "Hidden/veiled compassion" (semantic pair to Jion).
- **Modern Interpretations:** Sometimes linked to the same liturgical/temple naming stream as Jion/Jitte.
- **Conflicting Ideas & Origins:** Exact referent (temple/teacher/theme) debated in Shotokan notes.

The name Ji'in (慈陰) carries both linguistic and historical meaning, though its ambiguity has led to various interpretations. The first character, 慈 (Ji), represents qualities such as mercy, compassion, and love. The second character, 陰 (In), is more complex, symbolizing shadow, sanctuary, or ground. It also alludes to the concept of Yin from yin-yang philosophy, which signifies balance and harmony. Consequently, the name is often translated as "Temple Grounds," "Shadow of Mercy," or more provocatively, "Inverted Mercy."

The ambiguity surrounding the character 陰 has sparked debate; does it refer to a specific location, like temple grounds, or a spiritual concept that aligns with the idea of yin? The interpretation of "Inverted Mercy" is particularly fascinating, as it hints at a paradox at the heart of the kata: compassion is expressed through decisive, often violent, action. In a martial context, this could imply non-lethal subjugation, restraint, or protective violence performed in the service of peace.

To clarify the name and its connection to the "Jion group," Gichin Funakoshi proposed renaming the kata to Shokyo (松影), which translates to "Pine Shadow." However, this name did not gain popularity and ultimately failed to resonate with practitioners, allowing the original, enigmatic name to endure.

Ji'in's Historical Origins

The origins of Ji'in remain a mystery, and its creator is unknown. However, because of its similar opening salutation and structural features, Ji'in is often associated with the kata Jion and Jitte, suggesting a common origin or at least a shared transmission path. It likely emerged or was introduced during the late 18th or early 19th century, a time when Chinese martial arts were significantly influencing Okinawan traditions, particularly in the Tomari district.

The flowing techniques of the kata and Its distinctive Ming-style salutation, which features the left hand open over the right fist, suggest possible roots in ancient practices like Chinese temple boxing or Luohan Quan. However, some oral traditions indicate that Ji'in originated directly from the Tomari-te lineage, known for its agile and evasive techniques. The kata may represent a blend of various Chinese forms that were brought to Okinawa by early emissaries or monks. Nonetheless, it is important to note that, due to conflicting oral traditions and the lack of a definitive originator, the historical connections of Ji'in remain largely speculative and are based on educated guesses.

Despite this uncertainty, Gichin Funakoshi recognized the kata's importance and incorporated it into the early Shotokan curriculum, referencing it in his publications. Similarly, Anko Itosu may have contributed to the kata's preservation within the context of Tomari-te. Unfortunately, over time, Ji'in gradually lost formal recognition, leading to its marginalization in many modern martial arts curricula.

Applying Ji'in's Wisdom

Built on a foundation of diverse stances and principles that emphasize stability, balance, and adaptability, Ji'in utilizes Zenkutsu Dachi to project forward pressure and Kiba Dachi to establish power and facilitate smooth transitions. In some styles like Shito-ryu, Kokutsu Dachi is also used selectively. The kata's compact, multi-directional structure, combined with the frequent repetition of these stances, presents a unique challenge that demands both stability and endurance from the practitioner. It seems designed to refine a practitioner's timing, enhance defensive maneuvers, and develop internal balance, particularly under stress.

One of Ji'in's signature techniques is the Crossed Gedan-Uke, or lower block, performed with a distinctive hovering position. This versatile movement can suggest a sweep, jam, or entry into a trapping sequence. The kata also incorporates simultaneous defenses, featuring paired techniques that combine upper-level blocks with counterstrikes to address multiple or chained attacks. The frequent directional turns are crucial for defending against multiple opponents or for repositioning to disrupt an attacker's rhythm. Movements such as Kosa-Uke and unconventional strikes hint at deceptive entries into throws or pressure-point strikes, reflecting the close-range style characteristic of Tomari-te. The unique focus on striking high-level targets goes beyond mere blocking; it implies strategies for psychological disruption and feinting tactics.

Beyond the physical movements, Ji'in emphasizes internal principles. Practitioners are required to maintain emotional and mental composure even amidst chaotic directional changes. This focus on internal balance is particularly relevant during stationary sequences, where the concepts of rootedness and flow must coexist harmoniously. The principles of Control and Spiral Power are also essential, especially during turns that require a coiled preparation. This approach suggests that techniques should involve winding power into movements rather than relying solely on striking from a static position.

Ji'in's Diverse Paths

The history of Ji'in varies significantly among different karate styles. In Shotokan, the kata was introduced by Gichin Funakoshi during the early development of the style but was later removed from the Japan Karate Association (JKA) syllabus, contributing to its obscurity. In contrast, Shito-ryu has managed to preserve Ji'in, likely due to its connection to the Tomari-te lineage and its symbolic relationship with other kata such as Jion and Jitte. Ji'in also remains an advanced kata in several minor lineages, particularly within Wado-ryu and others.

These different lineages have led to notable stylistic variations. Shotokan practitioners typically employ a linear approach characterized by long stances and clear transitions. Shito-ryu, on the other hand, emphasizes faster directional changes, a variable tempo, and a sense of compression in its movements. Wado-ryu incorporates principles inspired by tuite, resulting in lighter and more fluid body mechanics.

Several factors contribute to these variations. Pedagogical drift has caused different styles to prioritize various teaching goals, leading some to retain Ji'in while others have discarded it based on perceived usefulness. As organizations like the JKA sought to streamline their curricula, Ji'in may have been removed to simplify testing standards or because it was seen as redundant due to its similarity to Jion.

While Ji'in itself has not given rise to new kata, it serves as an interpretive framework for understanding other forms like Jion and Jitte. This depth allows practitioners to gain insights into the structural and philosophical patterns within that group of kata. Legends and anecdotes further enrich its mystique. One theory suggests a connection to temple monks who utilized martial forms to protect sacred grounds, which is reflected in the interpretation of its name as "temple grounds." Another perspective posits that Ji'in may not have been its original designation, hinting at its true origins in Chinese secret societies or within family systems passed down orally through generations.

Ji'in's Lasting Impact

Ji'in is a kata that is often overlooked, yet it represents a subtle evolution within the temple kata group. Its origins are ambiguous, the naming is unusual, and the movement sequences are tightly wound. Practicing Ji'in requires nuanced control, patience, and a high degree of proprioceptive awareness. Despite its compressed form, it conceals a wealth of technical insights.

Although Ji'in is no longer part of the JKA's formal testing system, it remains an important kata for both historical continuity and technical refinement. For those looking to explore deeper layers within Okinawan and Japanese martial practices, Ji'in provides a glimpse into a less conventional aspect of kata; one that poses more questions than it answers but ultimately rewards the inquisitive with calm power and internal balance.

UNSHU

OKINAWA'S GATHERING STORM

Introduction to Unshu

Among the various kata practiced throughout Okinawa and Japan, few evoke as much technical intrigue and cultural confusion as Unshu; often referred to simply as Unsu in Japanese contexts. When you ask a Shotokan practitioner about Unsu, they may describe it as a spinning, high-kicking kata designed for tournament appeal. However, in Okinawa, where the form has deeper roots, Unsuu represents something entirely different: a storm of breath, body dynamics, and combat practicality. With origins traced back to the 19th-century master Aragaki Seisho and influenced by Southern Chinese boxing principles, Unsu warrants closer examination, particularly in its more grounded Okinawan variant.

This chapter will explore Unsu's original context, examining its name, history, mechanics, and philosophical meanings. We will contrast its Okinawan roots with its later evolution on the Japanese mainland and discuss why its cloud-like adaptability positions it as one of Okinawa's most sophisticated combative forms.

Exploring Unshu's Essence

- **Traditional Notation:** 雲手 (Unsu).
- **Script Breakdown:**
    - 雲 "cloud";
    - 手 "hand."
- **Core Meaning:** "Cloud hands."
- **Modern Interpretations:** Name evokes flowing, swirling handwork.
- **Conflicting Ideas & Origins:** Not contested; title appears descriptive.

The name Unsu (雲手) is made up of two kanji: 雲 (Un), meaning "cloud," and 手 (Shu), meaning "hand." Together, they create the term "Cloud Hands," a poetic and tactical metaphor that embodies the essence of the kata. In Okinawan dialects and early usage, the term was often pronounced as Unshu, while Unsu is the later Sino-Japanese reading that gained popularity through mainland systems like Shotokan and Shito-ryu.

Interestingly, there is a historical reference in a 1914 newspaper article that mentioned "舞手" (dance hand) and its pronunciation as "Unsu." This could possibly be a transcription error, but it supports the theory that Okinawan karate was influenced by the native dance known as Mekata. Gichin Funakoshi may have later chosen the more common kanji 雲手 ("Cloud Hand") for his 1922 book, making it easier for mainland readers to understand.

Interpretations of "Cloud Hands" vary. Some see the name as reflecting the kata's constant transitions, similar to how clouds form and reform in a turbulent sky, emphasizing shifting weight, spiraling limbs, and explosive movements. Others interpret it philosophically, linking it to the Zen concept of Hatsuun Jindo ("Parting the Clouds, Seeking the Way"), which suggests perseverance through obscurity. In both interpretations, the name captures the essence of a kata that is designed to be elusive yet powerful, unpredictable yet deeply principled.

Unshu's Historical Origins

The most credible link to the creation of Unshu points to Aragaki Seisho, an Okinawan diplomat, interpreter, and martial arts master skilled in Chinese systems such as White Crane and Monk Fist boxing. Serving the Shuri court during a time of increased contact between the Ryukyu Kingdom and China, Aragaki was well-positioned to absorb and transmit Chinese martial arts forms. It is believed that Unshu was either created by him or significantly adapted from Chinese source material under his guidance.

Although Aragaki was associated with the Shuri court, Unshu is more closely aligned with Naha-te traditions, suggesting either a regional blending of methods or a later integration into Naha-te lineages. Some Okinawan researchers argue that Unsu is a composite form, representing a sophisticated synthesis of techniques from various katas, including Kusanku, Bassai, Jion, Chintō, Jitte, Wanshu, and others. This would make Unsu a tactical summation; a form designed to integrate and refine techniques rather than merely to represent them.

Applying Unshu's Wisdom

The Okinawan variant of Unshu, particularly the Aragaki Unshu kata, emphasizes practical utility and internal control. Unlike the athletic jumping spin characteristic of the Shotokan version, this approach focuses on open-hand techniques such as ippon nukite, shuto, and elbow strikes known as hiji ate, along with palm deflections.

The kata incorporates dynamic transitions between stances, emphasizing neko-ashi-dachi and sanchin-dachi. These stances allow for rapid shifts between rooted and mobile postures, and allow the form to utilize coiling power, where the body loads and redirects energy through a spiraling motion; echoing principles found in Dragon-style kung fu. Additionally, there are numerous moments that highlight tuite potential, showcasing grappling techniques, seizing actions, and limb control, all consistent with traditional Okinawan methods.

Breath, timing, and internal tension play significant roles in this practice. Drawing from Naha-te's ibuki breathing, Unshu connects physical contraction and expansion with combative intent, enabling the practitioner to absorb, blend, and retaliate with precision. Rather than relying on linear, explosive power, the kata teaches how to enter an opponent's space, redirect momentum, and unbalance them through rotation.

Unshu's Diverse Paths

The kata Unsu became internationally recognized through Shotokan karate, but its Okinawan versions, often referred to as Aragaki Unshu, maintain a more practical and less stylized interpretation. This Okinawan lineage is relatively rare and is most commonly transmitted through Shito-ryu-derived schools or private dojos that uphold older teachings. The traditional form of Unsu is more grounded, less acrobatic, and focuses more on functional application than performance spectacle.

In mainland Japan, Unsu was adapted to be more stylized. It was introduced through Kenwa Mabuni's Shito-ryu and later incorporated into Gichin Funakoshi's Shotokan. The Shotokan version features a signature 360-degree spinning jump that includes a double kick, a visually striking movement not found in the traditional Okinawan practice. This stylistic shift reflects a focus on a more competitive environment and structured training, moving away from the interpretative, breath-guided motions of its original form.

Though Funakoshi first mentioned the kata in his 1922 book, "Ryukyu Kenpo Karate," there is no evidence that he learned it in its original context. It likely reached him through Mabuni or his contemporaries. Nevertheless, even in its Japanese variation, Unsu retains elements of its origins: swirling hand movements, deceptive footwork, and tactical misdirection remain central features. Both versions of Unsu represent different expressions of a common ancestor.

Additionally, another version of Unshu was passed down by Motobu Choyu, the older brother of Motobu Choki. This version, which still exists in Okinawa, represents a distinct lineage that may be connected to different influences.

Unshu's Lasting Impact

Unsu is a kata that embodies the essence of a storm; it represents turbulence with a core. In its Okinawan form, it showcases many ideals of advanced karate: adaptability, redirection, spiraling energy, and decisive control. This kata emphasizes the refinement of movement rather than mere flashy motions; it focuses on clarity of intent rather than choreography.

Influenced by Aragaki Seisho, Unsu serves as a connection between Southern Chinese martial theory and the practical realities of Okinawan combat. Its internal mechanics and strategic design provide insight into how Okinawan masters understood threats, timing, and control. Studying Unsu challenges not only one's technique but also one's mindset, promoting the ability to stay fluid, grounded, and purposeful under pressure.

To study Unsu is to learn how to clear the clouds, both literally and figuratively. For serious practitioners of Okinawan karate, it stands as a benchmark of martial sophistication: a gathering storm from which clarity and power emerge.

GOJUSHIHO
OKINAWA'S 54 FLOWS

Introduction to Gojushiho

To the casual observer, Gojushiho may seem alien; more akin to a coiled animal poised to strike than a traditional kata. Its movements are sharp, sinuous, and unpredictable. Featuring open-hand techniques that dart and twist, stances that slide rather than stomp, and transitions that flow like liquid across uneven ground, Gojushiho defies expectations. Even its name, which translates to "Fifty-Four Steps," does little to clarify the kata's deeper origins or purpose.

This chapter examines the complex lineage, intricate technical content, and often-overlooked cultural dimensions of Gojushiho, historically known as Useishi. Suspected to have roots in Chinese martial traditions and Okinawan court dances, Gojushiho has bifurcated into "Sho" and "Dai" variants in Japan. Rather than being a fixed kata, Gojushiho represents an evolving conversation passed down through generations.

Exploring Gojushiho's Essence

- **Traditional Notation:** 五十四歩 (Gojūshiho; dai/shō variants).
- **Script Breakdown:**
    - 五十 "50";
    - 四 "4"; 歩 "steps."
- **Core Meaning:** "54 steps."
- **Modern Interpretations:** Multiple long advanced versions; "steps" construed as counts/phases.
- **Conflicting Ideas & Origins:** Standardized title; lineage versions diverge.

Unlike many kata in the encyclopedia of Okinawan Karate, Gojushiho (五十四歩) has been recorded using kanji since its first appearances in writing. The name breaks down to "Go" (五, 5), "Ju" (十, 10), "Shi" (四, 4), and "Ho" (歩, steps or movements), literally translating to "Fifty-Four Steps." However, this number may not be arbitrary. In Buddhist-influenced systems, 54 and 108 hold spiritual significance; each is linked to cycles of purification, struggle, and enlightenment. Thus, some believe the number represents more than just a step count; it suggests a spiritual journey through martial cultivation.

Throughout its history, the kata has had many names. In Okinawa, it was referred to as "Useishi" (a phonetic rendering of the Chinese term for 54 movements) or "Sushiho." Gichin

Funakoshi attempted to rename it "Hotaku," meaning "woodpecker," in reference to the repeated pecking-like hand strikes, but the name did not gain widespread acceptance.

Today, Shotokan and some other styles feature two versions: Gojushiho Sho ("minor") and Gojushiho Dai ("major/greater"). Confusingly, in JKA tradition, the names were swapped from their original assignments, while SKIF and other organizations retained the older nomenclature. This inconsistency highlights the kata's fluid evolution across various systems.

Gojushiho's Historical Origins

The "Fifty-Four Steps" of Gojushiho stands as one of karate's most intricate and historically rich forms. Its roots stretch back to the early 19th century, or even earlier, considering its strong Chinese lineage. While Gojushiho did not appear prominently in public karate curricula until well after Itosu Anko's reforms, its complex nature likely meant it thrived primarily in private instruction, passed down only to serious students prepared for its sophistication. There's even an intriguing theory that the kata was based on, or at least influenced by Okinawan court dances, known as mēkata, performed at the Ryukyu royal court. This connection would position Gojushiho as one of the clearest bridges between Okinawan martial practice and its performative, aristocratic past.

The earliest documented Okinawan practitioner of Gojushiho was Yabu Kentsu, a product of both military rigor and classical training. Yabu learned the form in its Useishi variant, possibly from the lineage of Matsumura Sokon. Matsumura, a pivotal figure in Shuri-te, is often credited with introducing Gojushiho to Okinawa, allegedly having learned it from a Chinese military officer named Iwah in the 1820s. Matsumura's students, including Chogi Yoshimura, Chotoku Kyan, and Chomo Hanashiro, carried the kata forward, each subtly modifying it. Notably, Toyama Kanken preserved a distinct Koryu Useishi, said to be directly influenced by Yabu's version. Toyama's rendition was less linear, incorporating more circularity and softness, thereby retaining elements now lost in many modern Shotokan and contemporary interpretations.

Chinese influences are profoundly evident in both Gojushiho's body mechanics and rhythm. Scholars have linked it to forms described in the Chinese military compendium Wubei Zhi, especially those associated with Black Tiger or White Crane systems. The kata's characteristic open-hand postures, deceptive footwork, and strong emphasis on short-range striking distinctly echo southern Chinese fighting traditions. Furthermore, specific portions of the kata, particularly its angular foot placement and nukite techniques, find analogues in the Bubishi, further reinforcing its deep Chinese pedigree.

Despite its ancient origins, Gojushiho's integration into mainstream karate was a gradual process. Gichin Funakoshi, for instance, did not initially teach it upon his move to mainland Japan in 1922. It was only later, possibly influenced by Mabuni or Toyama, both of whom championed its depth, that he incorporated it, eventually developing the two modern Shotokan variants: Gojushiho Dai and Gojushiho Sho.

Applying Gojushiho's Wisdom

Gojushiho, unlike many other kata, is not a linear form; it flows and transitions between stances, reflecting a constant adaptation of weight, angle, and pressure. Its movements are primarily reactive rather than overtly assertive, meaning it does not push through opponents but rather moves around them. The kata also departs from a rigid tempo; some sequences explode into action while others deliberately hesitate, making timing a crucial tactical element. The transitions are remarkably subtle, featuring hidden steps, sliding shifts, and mid-motion adjustments that contribute to its elusive nature.

Gojushiho is renowned for its unorthodox strikes and versatile techniques. Among these are the versatile yonhon nukite, or four-finger spear hands, and the precise ippon nukite, characterized by one-finger thrusts. Its distinctive arsenal also includes "cane beak" strikes and circular shuto blocks that easily transition into parries or throws. In some versions, the opening techniques of Gojushiho notably resemble Aikido's flowing parries, with shifts in angle suggesting various entries and takedowns. Additionally, some sequences hint at throws, while others indicate potential eye gouges or clavicle strikes. The bunkai often explores practical scenarios, delving into sophisticated techniques such as weapon disarms, neck manipulations, and grappling in confined spaces.

What truly sets Gojushiho apart is its hallmark adaptability. If a particular movement proves ineffective, another follows smoothly in its place. This style embodies an exploratory energy, focusing less on executing a fixed attack and more on the guided unraveling of an opponent's structure. With its profound emphasis on close-range combat, Gojushiho cultivates heightened tactile sensitivity, precise breath coordination, and mental calmness amid rapid changes. Kime (focused energy) in Gojushiho is not about abruptly stopping movement; instead, it emphasizes a flowing resolution. Practitioners must internalize fluidity, becoming capable of crashing into an opponent like a wave or retreating like mist, demonstrating a profound command of dynamic balance and responsiveness.

Gojushiho's Diverse Paths

From Matsumura to Yabu, and onward to Hanashiro, Kyan, and Toyama, Gojushiho has branched widely. While it is found in many major styles today, its interpretations diverge dramatically.

Within the realm of karate, various stylistic variations showcase unique characteristics and approaches to movement. Shotokan, for instance, emphasizes the practice of Gojushiho Sho and Dai, known for its clean linear movements and distinct power generation. In contrast, Shito-ryu incorporates multiple versions of Gojushiho, merging elements from both the Tomari and Shuri lines to create a rich blend of techniques. Meanwhile, Toyama's Koryu Useishi features softer movements with layered applications, reflecting a different philosophy or approach to martial arts. Additionally, the Tomari-te versions sometimes portray swaying or off-balance postures, evoking the image of a "drunken man," which adds a unique dimension to their practice. Each of these styles contributes to the diverse landscape of karate, illustrating how tradition and technique can vary significantly within the discipline.

Differences stem from lineage, teaching goals, and regional emphasis. Some forms stress hard power, others subtlety and softness. Adaptations occurred when instructors adjusted the kata for sport, pedagogy, or to match the body dynamics of new generations.

Gojushiho's influence can be felt in advanced kata across systems. Its nuanced grasp of close-range dynamics and deceptive body movement has quietly informed the design of several modern bunkai sequences.

Gojushiho's Lasting Impact

Gojushiho is a kata characterized by whispers rather than declarations. It communicates through subtleties, such as the slide of a foot, the curve of a parry, and the gentle arc of a spear hand. Its name, "Fifty-Four Steps," suggests a structured path, but in reality, there is no fixed sequence in this form. Instead, it emphasizes choices, connections, and consequences.

Whether it originated from the Chinese Black Tiger style, Okinawan dance, or some now-forgotten Fujian system, Gojushiho remains a masterpiece of nuance. It does not demand brute strength; rather, it requires clarity, adaptability, and awareness. By mastering this kata, one learns not just a series of movements but also how to move with intention; quietly, effectively, and with unwavering focus.

ECHOES IN THE EMPTY HAND

Across these chapters, a pattern emerges, though it is not a linear one. The kata of Okinawan karate form a constellation rather than a hierarchy. Some kata are ancient forms passed down through fragmented lineages with unclear creators, while others are modern consolidations designed to organize curriculum or preserve elements of fading systems. Some kata are clearly combative, while others seem symbolic or didactic, masking their functionality behind rhythm and repetition. Each kata tells us something; not only about martial technique but also about the people and pressures that shaped it.

Several recurring themes are worth noting. First, the influence of Chinese systems, particularly from Fuzhou, is undeniable, although it is often generalized in Western accounts. This work aims to identify where specific Chinese principles (e.g., White Crane posture, Southern Tiger striking, Qinna-based grappling) likely entered Okinawan forms. Second, the use of numerical titles, such as Sanseru, Seisan, and Suparinpei, suggests not only mnemonic value but also deeper connections to Buddhist cosmology and body-based systems of categorization. Third, while many kata were adapted for public instruction in the twentieth century, their core mechanics still reflect a close-range, principle-based logic aligned with civilian self-protection; not tournament display or military formation.

Perhaps most importantly, kata as a training method survives because it is generative. No other training method in martial arts offers the same layered potential: solo practice, tactical sequencing, principle isolation, energy control, timing, and intent; all within a self-contained form. Properly understood, kata is not mere choreography; it is encoded decision-making.

As we transition into the second half, focused on kobudō kata, the reader will notice both continuity and contrast. Continuity in body mechanics, breathing, and close-quarters principles. Contrast in range, rhythm, and the use of tools that alter the nature of conflict. Nevertheless, the underlying thesis remains: each kata, whether weaponless or weaponed, contains a logic, a structure that, once deciphered, reveals far more than movement alone.

The first half has laid the groundwork. The second half will trace the weaponized extensions of these same principles, expressed not only through technique but also through timber, steel, and the ingenuity of a culture that found ways to transform necessity into mastery.

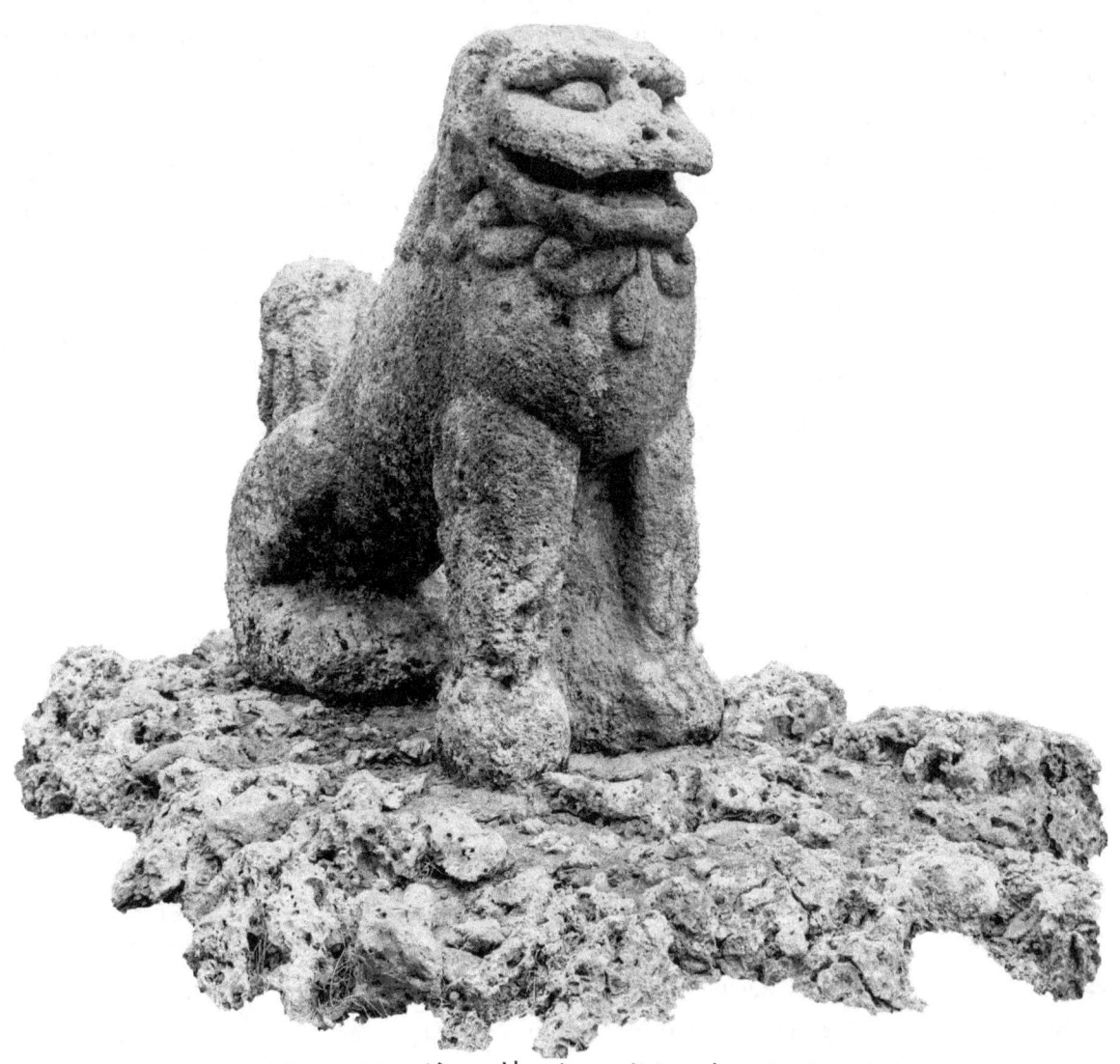

Tomori Stone Lion (シーサー), traditional protector statue
(April 2023)

BOOK TWO - KOBUDO KATA

OKINAWA'S WEAPONS: TRADITION IN TIMBER AND STEEL

If karate represents the empty hand of Okinawa, then kobudō serves as its armed counterpart. Both disciplines developed simultaneously, each preserving essential principles of distance, timing, and leverage, but expressing them in different ways. While empty-hand kata train the body as a weapon, kobudō kata extend those same mechanics into tools made of wood, iron, and cord; transforming everyday implements into instruments of survival and artistry.

The origins of Okinawan kobudō arise from a combination of necessity and creativity. Common tools, such as the bō (a carrying pole), the eku (an oar), the kama (a sickle), and the sai (a truncheon), were adapted into weapons due to local conflicts, foreign influences, and restrictions on arms. Over time, these adaptations were codified into kata, preserving not only combat techniques but also capturing the rhythms of Okinawa's working life and maritime culture. Therefore, studying kobudō kata offers insight into the pragmatism and creativity of the Ryukyu people.

However, these forms are not merely remnants of tools; they are dynamic systems. Kobudō kata require precision in managing unfamiliar weight and balance, enhancing the practitioner's awareness of range, rhythm, and intent. Just as empty-hand kata cultivate structure, breath, and spirit, weapon kata extend these qualities outward, demanding a harmonious integration between body and weapon. In doing so, they reveal the shared heritage of Okinawan martial traditions; common roots expressed through different branches.

In this section, we will explore the classical kobudō kata, examining their names, histories, lineages, and evolving interpretations. Some are linked to legendary figures like Chatan Yara or Tsuken Shitahaku, while others are associated with families or villages that still bear their names. Together, these kata represent not only a technical syllabus but also a cultural archive that records

Okinawa's resilience, its interactions with neighboring cultures, and the enduring spirit of innovation that transformed tools of labor into arts of defense.

SECTION I - BO-JUTSU KATA

OKINAWA'S STAFF: CARVING PATHS OF POWER

A simple wooden staff, typically about six feet long, the bō is one of the most iconic weapons in Okinawan kobudō. Its origins are sometimes connected to Chinese staff-fighting arts or to the poles used for carrying loads and navigating boats. However, in the context of Okinawan martial arts, the bō evolved into a versatile tool for both necessity and defense.

The bō exemplifies the Ryukyuan principle of transforming everyday objects into instruments of survival, turning a basic staff into a weapon for striking, blocking, sweeping, and leveraging. Within martial culture, it symbolizes both simplicity and sophistication, requiring mastery of distance, balance, and whole-body coordination. Often regarded as the "foundation weapon" of kobudō, the bō serves as a gateway to understanding the principles shared by other martial implements.

SAKUGAWA NO KUN
Okinawa's Staff Pioneer

Introduction to Sakugawa no Kun

When the name Sakugawa is mentioned in Okinawan martial arts circles, it represents not only a historical figure but also symbolizes evolution and transmission. Tode Sakugawa's legacy is one of quiet revolution, merging Chinese martial strategies with the unique culture of the Ryukyu Kingdom. His influence is perpetuated not through written records but in the dynamic movements of seasoned wood. "Sakugawa's Staff," or Sakugawa no Kun, embodies this legacy as one of the foundational kata in Okinawan kobudō, particularly in bojutsu.

Bearing the name of its creator, Sakugawa no Kun is a kata rich in technical significance and symbolic importance. It acts as a crucial link between the ancient Chinese staff systems that influenced early Okinawan fighting methods and the refined, codified forms that evolved within Ryukyu's martial culture. As a central component of the martial arts curriculum, studying this kata enables practitioners to connect with a historical lineage that stretches back to the origins of Okinawan kobudō.

This chapter will delve into the layered legacy of Sakugawa no Kun; its name, structure, philosophical roots, and technical sophistication. By examining the historical figure behind the kata and the principles embedded within the form, we will trace how this kata serves as both a physical curriculum and a symbolic link in the unbroken chain of Okinawan martial tradition.

Exploring the Essence of Sakugawa

- **Traditional Notation:** 佐久川の棍 (Sakugawa no Kon/Kun).
- **Script Breakdown:**
  - 佐久川 (Sakugawa, surname);
  - の possessive;
  - 棍 "staff."
- **Core Meaning:** "Sakugawa's staff form."
- **Modern Interpretations:** Attributed to the Sakugawa line (eponymic).
- **Conflicting Ideas & Origins:** Stable eponym; minor spelling variance (Kon/Kun) across sources.

The name "Sakugawa no Kun" holds significant meaning and is deeply rooted in the history of Okinawan martial arts. It can be broken down into three distinct parts, each reflecting the kata's origin and purpose. "Sakugawa" refers to Kanga "Tode" Sakugawa, a pivotal figure from the 18th century known for his contributions to the early integration of Chinese and Okinawan combative systems. The possessive particle "no," which translates to "of," serves as a connective element.

Finally, "Kun" is the Okinawan term for a six-foot-long staff, pronounced "bo" in Japanese. Together, these components honor Sakugawa and the martial tradition he helped shape.

While the name clearly points to the individual credited with creating or inspiring the kata, there is a historical debate among martial arts scholars and practitioners. This discussion revolves around whether the form practiced today is a direct artifact from Sakugawa himself or a later tribute created in his honor by subsequent generations. Some traditional schools claim to preserve an "older" version, believing it to have a more direct lineage from the master, while others acknowledge that their version is a more modern iteration, shaped through evolving bojutsu pedagogy and the teachings of later masters.

Attaching Sakugawa's name to a kata is not a casual act. In Okinawan martial tradition, this signifies not just respect but also a claim to a specific lineage and historical knowledge. This naming convention elevates the kata from being merely "a staff form" to being "his staff form," or one that directly reflects his principles. Therefore, the name functions as both a technical curriculum and a cultural vessel, distinguishing the kata as a crucial link in the historical chain of Okinawan kobudō.

Sakugawa no Kun's Historical Origins

The kata likely originated in the late 18th or early 19th century, during a time of significant Chinese cultural influence in the Ryukyu Kingdom. Its namesake was an important figure in this era, having studied martial arts under the Chinese military envoy Kusanku, and is widely recognized for his role in integrating Chinese martial concepts into Okinawan traditions. As the teacher of Matsumura Sokon, a foundational figure in modern karate and kobudō, Sakugawa's influence established a clear lineage that connects ancient practices to the present day.

The staff used in this kata was a common tool for Okinawan farmers, fishermen, and officials, making it a practical and accessible weapon. Due to restrictions on carrying bladed weapons imposed by Satsuma rule, the bo became codified into several family martial systems, to preserve and transmit combative techniques. Sakugawa no Kun functioned both as a teaching method and as a mobile record of movements that could endure over time. The kata's movements, which include its distinctive sweeping figure-eights and angular thrusts, seem to clearly show influence from Southern Chinese staff systems, particularly those from Fuzhou, which Sakugawa likely adapted for local use.

While earlier staff forms may have been practiced by court retainers or pechin guards, Sakugawa no Kun is significant as one of the first bojutsu kata formally associated with a named lineage. This established it not only as a technical curriculum but also as a historical link in the evolution of Okinawan martial tradition.

Applying Sakugawa's Combat Wisdom

A masterclass in foundational bojutsu principles, emphasizing a dynamic blend of rooted stability and fluid adaptability, Sakugawa no Kun's technical execution is built upon a strategic use of stances, each serving a distinct purpose.

The Zenkutsu Dachi is utilized for powerful, forward-driving thrusts and strikes, providing the necessary stability and momentum for a decisive attack. In contrast, the Neko Ashi Dachi, key for agile transitions, allows the practitioner to shift direction, retreat, or prepare for a deflection with speed and grace. The Hasso no Kamae (eight directions posture) serves as a technical centerpiece, facilitating a seamless flow between offensive and defensive movements. Even the kneeling Iaigoshi dachi is not a static poses but dynamic postures that form the foundation for effective combat strategies.

The techniques within the kata showcase a comprehensive approach to both offense and defense. Strikes demonstrate the use of powerful overhead and diagonal motions as well as precise head-level thrusts, designed to counter attacks from both armed and unarmed opponents. Blocks utilize cross-body and vertical motions, emphasizing the need for defense against long weapons and wide arcs of movement. The kata also incorporates leg-level sweeping motions to unbalance or trip an opponent, highlighting the importance of lower-body techniques in combat. A key element of the kata's technical depth is the focus on grip changes, where practitioners learn to adjust the length of the bo. This adaptability allows for a seamless transition between close-range and long-range techniques, a crucial skill for mastering distance control and spacing in weapon combat.

Beyond the visible techniques, the kata cultivates a number of internal principles essential to effective martial application. Power generation relies heavily on rotational torque, full-body coordination, and the snap generated by relaxed musculature. The rhythm of the kata is paramount; rushing breaks the form, while hesitation weakens intention. Ultimately, Sakugawa no Kun encourages a strong connection between grounding and reach, cultivating a unique blend of rooted stability and adaptable fluidity that defines Okinawan bojutsu.

Sakugawa's Diverse Paths

Sakugawa Kanga did not leave behind a written curriculum, but his teachings were preserved through his most famous student, Matsumura Sokon, and have since been passed down to various kobudō lineages. Today, the form known as Sakugawa no Kun can be found in multiple traditions, particularly within Ryukyu Kobudō, Ryu Kon Kai, Matsumura Seito, and other organizations dedicated to preserving classical Okinawan weapon systems. This history of transmission highlights the kata as a core component of bojutsu that has survived for centuries through oral tradition and practical practice.

Due to this long history of transmission through different masters and schools, significant stylistic variations of the kata have emerged. Differences can be observed in the kata's tempo, the total number of techniques, and the direction of movements. Some older versions are often simpler and more linear, while others have incorporated flashier spins and embellishments, likely due to influences from modern, competition-oriented systems. These variations are not flaws but rather hallmarks of Okinawan practice; they reflect each lineage's philosophical emphasis, whether it be on practicality, beauty, or complexity. This fluidity illustrates how the kata has evolved through pedagogical adaptation, stylistic focus, and the personal interpretations of successive masters.

As one of the oldest named bo kata in Okinawan kobudō, Sakugawa no Kun serves as a foundational blueprint for many other staff forms. Its movements and core principles resonate throughout other kata, such as Shushi no Kun and Choun no Kun, suggesting that Sakugawa's influence extends well beyond a single form.

The Enduring Legacy of Sakugawa

In the practice of Okinawan bojutsu, Sakugawa no Kun is not merely a sequence of staff techniques; it embodies a philosophy and serves as a mobile archive of movement, representing a pivotal moment in martial history. This kata showcases the successful adaptation of Chinese martial strategies into a distinctly Okinawan form, rooted in practical combat and enhanced through disciplined practice. Every movement—whether it involves subtle grip adjustments or powerful sweeping arcs—imparts fundamental lessons in economy, distance, rhythm, and power.

Ultimately, the enduring legacy of this kata lies in its nature as a living artifact. Each time it is practiced, the influence of Tode Sakugawa resonates through generations. His contributions serve as a bridge between Chinese and Okinawan cultures, between empty-hand techniques and weaponry, and between the secrecy of earlier methods and the structured pedagogy of kata. Sakugawa no Kun reminds us that in Okinawan kobudō, a staff is never just a stick; it is a legacy in motion.

SHUSHI NO KUN

Okinawa's Flowing Staff Lineage

Introduction to Shushi no Kun

It's easy to overlook Shushi no Kun as just another bo kata. Unlike Sakugawa no Kun, which has broader name recognition, Shushi no Kun lacks flashy movements often seen in modern competitive forms. However, beneath its fluid sweeps and precise deflections lies a story that dates back nearly two centuries to a Chinese master teaching staff techniques in the backstreets of Naha. Shushi no Kun, which translates to "Mr. Shu's Staff," is a foundational kata in Okinawan kobudō. Although it appears simple on the surface, its elegant design makes it one of the first forms taught in Yamane-ryu and various other traditional bojutsu lineages. This kata not only serves as an introduction to staff combat for many, but also provides insight into the deep cultural and martial exchange between Okinawa and China.

This chapter delves into the historical legacy, linguistic nuances, technical construction, and variations in lineage associated with Shushi no Kun. We will illustrate how a kata with Chinese roots became a cornerstone of Okinawa's unique weapons tradition.

Unveiling Shushi no Kun's Essence

- **Traditional Notation:** 周氏の棍 (Shūshi no Kun).
- **Script Breakdown:**
  - 周氏 "Mr. Zhou/Chō (Shushi)" (surname + clan marker);
  - の possessive;
  - 棍 "staff."
- **Core Meaning:** "Mr. Zhou's staff form."
- **Modern Interpretations:** Eponymic title preserved across Ryūkyū kobudō lines.
- **Conflicting Ideas & Origins:** Which historical "Shushi" is referenced varies in oral accounts.

The name "Shushi no Kun" (周氏の棍) has significant meaning that directly connects the kata to its historical origins. It consists of three distinct components. "Shushi" (周氏) is the Japanese pronunciation of the Chinese surname Zhou, and with the honorific suffix, it translates to "Mr. Zhou" or "Mr. Shu." The possessive particle "no" (の) means "of" and links the name to the weapon. Lastly, "Kun" (棍) is the Okinawan term for the six-foot staff weapon, which is known as "bo" in Japanese martial arts. Together, these elements create the title "Mr. Shu's Staff," paying homage to a figure whose identity is central to the kata's history.

While the name may seem straightforward, its implications are layered. The use of a Chinese name for the kata clearly indicates that its origin is not Okinawan, but rather imported, studied, and preserved. Whether the person's name was truly Shu (Zhou) or if this was a symbolic name remains a subject of historical debate. Regardless, the name itself is a profound act of cultural significance. In Okinawan martial culture, naming a kata after a person is a powerful way to acknowledge lineage and connect the art to its origins. "Shu" becomes more than just a teacher's name; it symbolizes the substantial influence from the Chinese mainland, representing a cultural fingerprint embedded in Okinawa's kobudō tradition.

Shushi no Kun's Historical Roots

The historical origins of Shushi no Kun are a fascinating blend of oral tradition and martial lineage, highlighting a period of significant cultural exchange between Okinawa and China. The kata's namesake, "Mr. Shu" (or Zhou), is traditionally believed to have been a Chinese martial artist from Shanghai who lived behind the Sogenji temple in Naha's Asato district around 1831. According to this widely accepted oral history, he taught this staff form to his Okinawan students. Although details about him are scarce, his legacy lives on in the kata itself.

However, historical accounts are not entirely consistent. Some researchers, including those cited in the *Bugei Ryuha Daijiten*, attribute the creation of the kata to a noble from Shuri and a bojutsu master named Soeishi. This theory suggests that the Soeishi family, who served as martial arts instructors to the Ryukyu king, developed the kata as part of their secret bojutsu tradition.

Despite these differing accounts, two key figures stand out in the formalization and dissemination of Shushi no Kun in Okinawa. The first is Chinen Sanda, a member of the Pechin class who studied various weapon teachings. He is recognized for his three bojutsu kata, including Shushi no Kun, and his transmission of these techniques to his son, Masami Chinen, laid the foundation for what would become the Yamane-ryu lineage. The second significant figure is the aforementioned Chinese master, Shu, who may have contributed to the development of the techniques that would eventually be recognized as Shushi no Kun.

Whether introduced by a Chinese master or developed by an Okinawan noble, the kata's structure and characteristics strongly suggest its introduction in the early 1830s. This was a period marked by robust cultural exchange with China, particularly in the ports of Naha and Tomari. Stylistically, the kata aligns with Southern Chinese gunshu (staff) systems, which emphasize close-quarters engagement, sweeping attacks, and rooted power. This indicates a direct influence from Fuzhou and other Southern Chinese traditions.

Shushi no Kun likely served both practical and educational purposes. Its techniques are accessible to beginners yet rich in subtlety, making it an ideal choice for early instruction while still allowing for deep refinement over time. Additionally, the kata provided a means for Okinawans to internalize and honor valuable foreign martial knowledge, establishing it as a foundational element in the evolution of Okinawan bojutsu.

Applying Shushi no Kun's Combat Wisdom

The kata Shushi no Kun is a masterclass in economy and fluid movement, built on principles that emphasize rotational power and strategic positioning. The form utilizes foundational stances like Zenkutsu-dachi but frequently transitions into narrower, more mobile positions that prioritize agility. One of the kata's defining principles is the continuous engagement of the hips; almost every block and strike is rooted in hip rotation, providing both stability and torque. A characteristic footwork pattern often involves the right foot subtly dropping away—a seemingly passive retreat that is actually a strategic repositioning to gain a structural advantage for a counterattack.

The techniques and bunkai of this kata are designed to be both efficient and deceptive. Defense does not rely on hard blocks but instead focuses on "receiving" deflections that absorb and redirect an opponent's force, buying a crucial moment to prepare for a counterattack. Sweeps and low strikes are vital components, targeting the knees and ankles to destabilize an attacker and disrupt their balance. Additionally, precise thrusts and pokes aimed at vulnerable areas highlight the pragmatic, real-world applications of these techniques. Rotational defense is also crucial, with the bo moving in small circles to redirect strikes while simultaneously setting up the next movement.

Beyond the physical aspects, Shushi no Kun is an exercise in internal control and focused intention. It demands an economy of motion, ensuring that nothing is wasted. The concepts of muchimi (stickiness or heaviness) and rootedness are heavily emphasized, particularly when transitioning or receiving force. The circular motion of the bo requires a relaxed upper body and an engaged core, allowing for sensitivity to an opponent's movements while delivering rapid, focused power. In this kata, every strike is paired with breath, posture, and focus (kime), highlighting that intention is as important as the physical impact itself.

Shushi no Kun's Evolving Traditions

Shushi no Kun has a rich history of transmission that has shaped its modern variations. Its journey likely began with a mysterious Chinese instructor in 1831 and was later formalized by Chinen Sanda, making the kata a foundational element of Yamane-ryu. Through the influence of Matsumura Sokon and Chinen's ongoing legacy, the principles of Shushi no Kun branched out into other kobudō traditions.

One of the most notable aspects of the kata's evolution is the existence of significant stylistic variations. Some lineages practice both Shushi no Kun Sho (minor) and Shushi no Kun Dai (major). These versions differ in length, complexity, and technical emphasis. While Yamane-ryu typically teaches the Sho version as a foundational form, other systems may choose to begin with the Dai version or treat both as distinct expressions of the same underlying principles.

These variations highlight the organic nature of Okinawan martial arts, where a master's personal interpretation, pedagogical adaptation, and stylistic emphasis all contribute to a kata's evolution. A teacher might adjust the tempo or posture to better suit a student's needs or to emphasize specific combat scenarios. While some systems favor a more linear approach, others explore the circularity of techniques. This fluidity is a hallmark of a living tradition; the core remains the same, but the branches diverge.

As one of the earliest named bojutsu katas, Shushi no Kun has played a significant role in defining Yamane-ryu's focus on hip-powered strikes and circular motion. Its principles can be seen echoed in other Okinawan bo forms, such as Choun no Kun and Sakugawa no Kun, serving as both a conceptual relative and potentialy a derivative.

Shushi no Kun's Lasting Impact

In the practice of Okinawan bojutsu, Shushi no Kun is more than just a kata; it represents a chapter in the centuries-long dialogue between Okinawa and China. This kata embodies a philosophy of combat that is both practical and elegant, teaching practitioners to utilize circular motion, hip-driven power, and adaptive defense. The fluid transitions, soft blocks, and powerful sweeps in the kata may seem deceptively simple, yet they conceal a profound depth of combative strategy.

Today, Shushi no Kun is practiced across various Okinawan kobudō systems and remains a rite of passage for bo practitioners, particularly in Yamane-ryu and beyond. It serves as a living reminder that within a simple piece of wood, one can discover a rich lineage, the power of adaptation, and an enduring legacy. Whether you learn the Sho (minor) or Dai (major) version, the kata resonates with the gentle voice of a foreign master as well as the resilient spirit of Okinawan martial tradition.

Choun no Kun

Okinawa's Sweeping Staff Strategy

Introduction to Choun no Kun

For many practitioners, Choun no Kun is often encountered after becoming familiar with the fundamentals of Shushi no Kun and Sakugawa no Kun. However, within its sweeping arcs, angled thrusts, and demanding rhythm lies a kata that, while seemingly straightforward, requires much more from the student than just muscle memory. Its name, a topic of debate and speculation, raises questions about its origins and historical significance.

Choun no Kun is a dynamic and technically rich bo kata practiced across several major Okinawan kobudō traditions. Known for its flowing combinations, deep stances, and tactical engagement with timing and distance, it serves as a bridge between foundational forms and more advanced combat principles. Although the movements may seem relatively simple at first glance, executing them properly demands a high degree of precision, sensitivity, and awareness.

This chapter will explore the intriguing complexities of Choun no Kun, covering its disputed origins, technical mechanics, strategic underpinnings, and its role in shaping the modern kobudō curriculum. We will examine the interpretive flexibility that continues to make it a central kata in the practice of Okinawan weapons.

Unveiling Choun no Kun's Essence

- **Traditional Notation:** (Varies) 長恩の棍 is sometimes seen; also "Chōun" as a nickname; orthography not uniform.
- **Script Breakdown:**
  - If 長恩: 長 "long/chief";
  - 恩 "favor"—but many write it in kana to avoid false precision.
- **Core Meaning:** "Chōun's staff."
- **Modern Interpretations:** Eponymic; often taught alongside Shushi/Sakugawa lines.
- **Conflicting Ideas & Origins:** Kanji differ among schools; often left in katakana.

The name "Choun no Kun" is both historically and linguistically intriguing. Typically rendered in Katakana as チョウンの棍, the name's construction suggests a non-Japanese origin. The first part, "Choun" (チョウン), is likely a transliteration of a Chinese name, possibly referring to a historical figure or a legendary character. The possessive particle "no" (の) serves as a link, while "Kun" (棍) is the Okinawan term for a traditional six-foot staff. Together, the name translates to "Choun's Staff," a seemingly simple title with a rich and complex history.

There is an ongoing debate about the identity of "Choun." Some believe it refers to a specific but now obscure Chinese martial artist whose teachings influenced a particular lineage. Others suggest a more romantic interpretation, linking the name to "Zhao Yun" (趙雲), the famed general from the Chinese historical novel *Romance of the Three Kingdoms*, known in Japanese as Choun. While this connection may be more folkloric than factual, it highlights the cultural and literary influences that permeated Okinawan society. Another theory links the name to a warrior from the Tomari area of Okinawa, though this remains speculative.

Regardless of its exact origin, the name "Choun no Kun" underscores a broader truth about Okinawan martial arts: they are deeply influenced by Chinese traditions, not just in technique but also in their naming, framing, and pedagogy. The kata's Chinese-sounding name preserves this lineage in linguistic form, acting as a cultural fingerprint that points to origins beyond the Ryukyu Islands.

Choun no Kun's Historical Roots

While the specific origin of Choun no Kun remains a topic of considerable debate in Okinawan kobudō, its historical significance is undeniable. Some lineages attribute the kata to an influential but unidentified Chinese martial artist who impacted Okinawan bojutsu during the late 18th or early 19th century. This theory aligns with the kata's name and the known cultural exchange between Okinawa and China during that period. Others propose that the kata was developed within Okinawan martial circles in Shuri, or possibly even Tomari, and was later named in honor of a Chinese figure or influence.

What is more certain is the kata's place in modern history. The earliest consistent references to Choun no Kun appear in the late 19th to early 20th century, aligning its formal transmission with the broader codification of karate and kobudō in Okinawa. It became part of the modern curriculum through prominent schools like Matayoshi Kobudō, Yamane-ryu, and various lineages influenced by Shinken Taira, passed down by senior teachers dedicated to preserving traditional weapon forms.

Stylistically, Choun no Kun exhibits the clear characteristics of Southern Chinese staff techniques, featuring short bursts of power, angular thrusts, and dynamic redirection. It likely serves as a bridge between beginner and advanced forms, allowing students to refine their fundamentals while introducing more complex timing, angles, and footwork. Its sequences balance offense and defense, creating a tight interplay ideal for teaching flow, rhythm, and reactive combat logic. This emphasis on control and targeting also parallels several Okinawan empty-hand kata in its combative intent.

Applying Choun no Kun's Combat Wisdom

The kata Choun no Kun is a dynamic exploration of foundational bojutsu principles, requiring both stability for powerful forward drives and fluid motion for agile transitions and evasive maneuvers. Proper weight shifting is crucial, especially during the pivots, drops, and forward movements that define its rhythm. Each technique begins with structural integrity and ends with kinetic intention, emphasizing that power is generated from the ground up.

The footwork in this kata is particularly demanding, requiring conscious engagement. The pivoting actions and angular changes simulate evasive movements while allowing the practitioner to maintain forward pressure. The right foot often takes on a mobile role, but it is the hips that initiate nearly all power, a principle known in Okinawan martial arts as gamaku (hip control).

The techniques themselves demonstrate a masterclass in dynamic, offensive-minded combat. Head and mid-level strikes are delivered in rapid succession, mimicking responses to both vertical and horizontal attacks while maintaining relentless forward pressure. The kata also features double blocks; a powerful and strategic defensive maneuver, not merely a passive deflection, it actively redirects the opponent's weapon or limb, creating an opening for a counter-attack or enabling a follow-up technique. Additionally, scooping motions, which can be interpreted as leg sweeps, disarms, or movements that enable low-line attacks, play a crucial role in the flow of the kata.

A vital aspect of these techniques is the use of kiai at key moments of decisive action. These are typically executed during a final thrust or a committed block-counter sequence. The kiai not only marks physical exertion but also signals a psychological climax, reinforcing the intensity and focus required in a combative engagement.

Beyond the physical movements, Choun no Kun cultivates various internal principles. Muchimi is essential; it helps keep the bo in motion and "connected" to both the practitioner's body and intent. Transitions are not pauses but rather pivots, and turns are not retreats but setups for future movements. Over time, students learn to sense the rhythm of the kata, allowing it to evolve from a mechanical performance into a fluid, combative conversation.

Choun no Kun's Evolving Traditions

The kata Choun no Kun holds a prominent place in the curricula of several major kobudō systems, a testament to its enduring value. It is particularly important within Matayoshi Kobudō, where it forms a foundational trio alongside Shushi no Kun and Sakugawa no Kun. Here, the kata emphasizes strong stances, powerful strikes, and the use of wrist rotations. A distinctive feature is the "double block," a strategic technique designed to maximize contact and redirect an opponent's attack.

In Yamane-ryu and Yamanni-Chinen-ryu, the kata is also taught, sometimes in two variations: Choun no Kun Sho and Choun no Kun Dai. The Yamane-ryu version is typically shorter and emphasizes fluid, dynamic movements, with a focus on continuous flow and rhythm. The goal is to make the body and the bo move as one, a hallmark of the style. Additionally, within the Taira Shinken and Ryukyu Kobudō Hozon Shinko Kai traditions, Choun no Kun is presented in both standard and old style versions, reflecting the diverse interpretations that can exist even within a unified system.

These stylistic variations arise from several factors, including the pedagogical filtering of different combative principles and the personal interpretations of master instructors. The kata's evolution has also been shaped by its performance context, moving from battlefield simulations to dojo instruction over the years. These differences are not a flaw but a reflection of the fluid nature of a living martial art. While the root remains the same, each lineage adapts the form to suit its own teaching methods, training goals, and stylistic emphasis.

While Choun no Kun is not usually cited as a parent kata, its techniques have profoundly influenced the broader strategy of Okinawan bo work. Its principles of transitional movement, control, and precise timing in mid-range weapon engagements are echoed in other bo forms, showcasing its lasting impact on the art.

The Lasting Impact of Choun no Kun

In the practice of Okinawan kobudō, Choun no Kun stands out as a crucial kata; not due to its complexity, but because of the fundamental mastery it requires from the practitioner. It demands precision without tension, rhythm without rigidity, and power without wasted motion. While the specifics of its lineage may be debated, its value as a teaching tool is unquestionable.

Dojo practitioners around the world continue to use Choun no Kun to test and refine serious students. This kata rewards patience and punishes shortcuts, encouraging practitioners to develop a deeper connection between their bodies and their weapons. Its flowing movements, clean lines, and emphasis on practical application have solidified its status not only as a transitional form but also as a standard for what a bo kata should embody: it is combative, cultural, and complete.

TOKUMINE NO KUN

Okinawa's Noble Guardian of the Staff

Introduction to Tokumine no Kun

In Okinawa's martial history, certain figures are remembered for their political influence, while others are celebrated for their martial skills. Tokumine Peichin is notable for being both. After being exiled to the remote Yaeyama Islands due to a political offense, he brought with him a mastery of the six-foot staff, which over time evolved into one of kobudō's most respected kata.

Tokumine no Kun is distinguished among Okinawan bo forms not only for its technical depth but also for the vibrant personality behind its name. Its sweeping arcs, controlled thrusts, and refined footwork combine battlefield practicality with the personal style of a skilled fighter who adapted to life far from the political center of Shuri. Today, it is practiced in various kobudō systems, most notably in Isshinryu Karate, where Tatsuo Shimabuku regarded it as his favorite kata.

This chapter will explore the historical roots of Tokumine no Kun, tracing its connection to Tokumine Peichin's exile. We will examine the kata's unique technical and strategic qualities and follow its journey through different lineages into the modern era. Additionally, we will consider its philosophical significance as a living link between political upheaval, cultural adaptation, and the preservation of martial traditions.

Exploring Tokumine no Kun's Essence

- **Traditional Notation:** 徳嶺の棍 (Tokumine no Kun).
- **Script Breakdown:**
    - 徳嶺 "Tokumine" (Pēchin Tokumine);
    - の possessive;
    - 棍 staff.
- **Core Meaning:** "Tokumine Pēchin's staff."
- **Modern Interpretations:** A signature bō form associated with Tokumine lineage.
- **Conflicting Ideas & Origins:** Name and translation are fairly set.

The name Tokumine no Kun holds deep cultural and historical significance. It consists of three parts: "Tokumine" (徳嶺), a family name made up of two kanji characters: "徳" (toku), meaning "virtue," and "嶺" (mine), meaning "ridge" or "peak." This combination evokes a sense of moral excellence associated with a high place. The possessive particle "no" (の) translates to "of," linking the name to the weapon, while "Kun" (棍) is the Okinawan term for the six-foot staff known as Bo in Japanese. Together, the name translates to "The Bo of the Tokumine Family," honoring both the individual and his lineage.

There is no doubt that the name refers to the historical figure Tokumine Peichin. However, the discussion among martial arts scholars centers on whether the kata as we know it today is a direct and unaltered artifact from his time or a form adapted by later instructors. Some researchers argue that Tokumine refined and reorganized techniques he encountered locally, such as the Akahachi no Bo forms from the Yaeyama Islands, which influenced the kata's content. Accounts placing Tokumine in a period of relative isolation suggest he may have adapted preexisting island techniques into a distinctive and portable curriculum that later teachers codified and standardized. By naming the kata after its originator, Okinawan martial tradition does more than just preserve a technical sequence; it honors the life and circumstances of a skilled martial artist who brought his art into isolation.

Tokumine no Kun's Historical Roots

The kata directly connects to the life of its namesake, Tokumine Peichin, who was a member of the pechin class, the warrior-bureaucrats of the Ryukyu Kingdom. Accounts vary regarding the precise reason for his exile, but it is widely believed that he was sent to the remote Yaeyama Islands for a political offense, either due to overstepping his authority or clashing with higher-ranking officials.

His exile likely occurred in the mid-to-late 19th century, a tumultuous period in Okinawa, following the Satsuma occupation and preceding the formal dissolution of the Ryukyu Kingdom. While in Yaeyama, Tokumine encountered local bo traditions, particularly those associated with the legendary figure Akahachi. It is believed that he synthesized these influences with his prior training from the Shuri martial arts circles to create a new kata. This blending of styles is evident in the kata's sweeping, circular movements and thrusting techniques, which demonstrate clear influences from Yaeyama Bojutsu and even Sojutsu (spear fighting).

For Tokumine, developing and refining this kata likely served as a means of personal discipline and a way to preserve his martial identity while in isolation. The structure of the kata reflects not only combat practicality but also distills his experiences into moves that are efficient, adaptable, and rooted in the realities of Okinawan and Yaeyama weapon encounters. The rhythmic quality and emphasis on control and precision in Tokumine no Kun echo his Shuri-based training, making it a unique and multifaceted martial artifact.

Applying Tokumine no Kun's Combat Wisdom

The kata Tokumine no Kun showcases dynamic and multifaceted bojutsu, built on a foundation of both stability and fluid evasion. The form consistently balances committed, linear power with agile repositioning, measured shifts, pivots, and periodic advances and retreats, allowing for rapid redirection and control of distance. A defining principle is that balance is never sacrificed for reach; every thrust originates from the hips and maintains centered alignment, ensuring that both power and recoverability remain consistent, even during extended techniques.

The kata organizes a small set of interlocking technical strategies into an efficient combat system. Circular sweeps serve as practical tools to deflect, unbalance, or redirect an opponent's bo and create openings for counterattacks. Complementing these sweeps are spiral or twisting thrusts, where a subtle rotation of the hands and hips enhances penetration while stabilizing the body during the attack.

Cross-body blocks play a dual role, simultaneously protecting high and low lines while setting up ripostes, allowing defense and offense to flow seamlessly into one another. The influence of spear fighting is evident in the spear-like lunges that quickly close the distance, delivering long-reaching thrusts to surprise an opponent. The kata emphasizes 45-degree angle entries to highlight the importance of attacking from unexpected angles to increase the likelihood of a successful engagement.

Ultimately, the core principles and techniques of Tokumine no Kun demonstrate a comprehensive strategy that blends the practicality of Okinawan bojutsu with a unique and refined fighting sensibility.

Tokumine no Kun's Evolving Traditions

The transmission of Tokumine no Kun is a prime example of how Okinawan weapon arts transitioned from local practice to broader circulation while maintaining their regional character. This form is credited to Tokumine Peichin and was introduced into the wider Okinawan tradition by Kyan Chotoku, who reportedly learned it during his travels to the Yaeyama Islands, where Tokumine had been exiled. Kyan's adoption of the kata and his subsequent teaching helped integrate this island-derived material into the Shuri–Naha training networks, from which it spread throughout the 20th century.

One of the most significant factors contributing to the kata's modern popularity was Tatsuo Shimabuku, who studied under Kyan and later included Tokumine no Kun in the Isshinryu kobudō curriculum. Shimabuku frequently cited it as one of his favorite weapons kata and played a crucial role in its mainstream transmission. His interpretation emphasized compact, powerful movements and clear angular shifts, which aligned with Isshinryu's practical approach focused on economy of motion. Conversely, other prominent kobudō teachers maintained their own versions: lineages associated with Shinken Taira and Matayoshi Shinko have variants that feature different embusen, timing, and technical focuses. In contrast, teachers connected to Matsumura-seito traditions, often represented by conservative lineages such as those linked with Hohan Soken and Kise Fusei, prioritize strict preservation of older Okinawan methods rather than adapting them for modern sport.

Stylistically, the variations are distinctive yet complementary. The Isshinryu version is generally compact and direct, emphasizing strong linear strikes and sharp transitions. Taira-influenced versions tend to be more expansive, favoring extended circular movements and fluid connections between techniques. The variants from Yaeyama preserve a particularly sweeping, almost dance-like quality, reflecting their island cultural roots and the local bojutsu aesthetics that inspired Tokumine.

Tokumine no Kun's Lasting Impact

Tokumine no Kun is best understood as a dynamic narrative: a concise martial biography shaped by Tokumine Peichin's journey from the administrative and martial culture of Shuri to enforced residence in the Yaeyama Islands. This social and geographic displacement, combined with his status as a Pechin, helped forge a martial form that emerged in isolation while being influenced by local island bojutsu. As a result, the kata reflects both personal circumstances and regional techniques.

Technically, the form distills practical bojutsu into a few interlocking principles. It emphasizes rooted forward power and hip-driven thrusts for stability and penetration, while narrower transitional stances and flexible footwork facilitate pivots, rapid redirections, and maintenance of tactical distance. Circular sweeps disrupt an opponent's structure and create openings, while spiral or twisting thrusts blend torque and stability for decisive finishing strikes. Cross-body blocks protect multiple lines and can quickly transition to counters, while spear-like lunges take advantage of reach and timing. When trained attentively, these elements demonstrate how balance, connection, and efficiency of movement govern the kata's applications.

The kata's transmission history emphasizes its dual nature as both a practical method and a cultural artifact. Kyan Chotoku is credited with bringing the form from Yaeyama to the Shuri-Naha networks. His students, particularly Tatsuo Shimabuku, carried and codified the kata into modern curricula, elevating it within Isshinryu and popularizing a compact, direct interpretation. Concurrent preservations by instructors from the Taira, Matayoshi, and Matsumura-seito lineages produced stylistic variations: longer, more flowing island renditions, broader Taira versions, and conservative preserves; each shaped by different teaching methods, body types, and audiences. These variations complement rather than contradict one another, as they retain the kata's core tactical logic while reflecting local aesthetics. Tokumine no Kun's significant contribution to Okinawan bojutsu is the integration of spear techniques into staff work, a legacy evident across multiple lineages.

TSUKEN NO KUN

Okinawa's Island Way of the Staff

Introduction to Tsuken no Kun

There's a certain elegance in the way Tsuken no Kun flows; a dance of the bo that conceals lethal intent behind circular grace. To the untrained eye, it might look like little more than a sequence of spins, thrusts, and steps. To those who know its history, each movement carries the weight of generations, the memory of a small Okinawan community, and the precision of a craftsman's tool honed for survival.

 In the Matayoshi Kobudō tradition, Tsuken no Kun is more than a technical exercise; it is a living record of the island's coastal warrior heritage. This chapter will explore its linguistic origins, the layered history of its transmission, the combat principles embedded in its form, and its evolution within the Matayoshi system.

Exploring Tsuken no Kun's Essence

- **Traditional Notation:** 津堅の棍 (Tsuken no Kun).
- **Script Breakdown:**
    - ○津堅 "Tsuken" (island/toponym);
    - ○の posessive;
    - ○棍 staff.
- **Core Meaning:** "Tsuken-island staff form."
- **Modern Interpretations:** Sometimes called **Chikin Bo** in Okinawan reading.
- **Conflicting Ideas & Origins:** Multiple Tsuken bō kata existed by 1930s; names overlap.

Tsuken no Kun (津堅の棍) literally translates to "the bo of Tsuken." The name "Tsuken" refers to Tsuken-jima, a small island off the eastern shore of Okinawa. The kanji 津 (tsu) typically denotes a harbor or ferry landing, while 堅 (ken) conveys meanings of firmness or solidity; however, in this context, they primarily serve as phonetic characters representing the island's name. The particle の (no) denotes possession, translating to "of," and 棍 (kun) refers to a long wooden staff, or bo. Therefore, the full phrase identifies both the implement and its geographic origin.

Like many kata names in Okinawa, Tsuken no Kun functions as both a geographic and cultural label, as well as a technical one. Locally, the name can indicate a form developed on Tsuken, a style associated with the island, or a sequence linked to a prominent teacher from Tsuken. Oral traditions often attribute its origin to a notable local master, commonly known as Chikin Kraka or Tsuken Mantaka. Other accounts suggest that the form represents a codification of a community-wide bojutsu practice.

Consequently, the nomenclature serves multiple cultural purposes: it grounds the kata in a specific place and community, preserves the memory of lineage, whether communal or individual, and signals a distinct regional aesthetic within Okinawan kobudō. However, the geographic name does not guarantee a single, unchanging technique; variations among teachers and lineages are common. Thus, the title points practitioners toward a shared origin and identity while also accommodating stylistic differences.

Tsuken no Kun's Historical Roots

The kata Tsuken no Kun emerged from the practical needs of a small maritime community on Tsuken Island. Here, fishermen and boatmen transformed everyday tools like boat poles and oars into effective weapons. These "fisherman-warriors" developed compact, reliable techniques tailored for the confined spaces of decks and docks, where sudden confrontations were common. The kata's movements and purpose are a direct reflection of this lived environment.

Attribution for this martial form relies more on local tradition and familial lineage than on written records. Oral histories trace the kata back through generations of Tsuken masters, whose collective practices were later preserved by named instructors. For instance, the Matayoshi kobudō lineage traces its Tsuken Bo back to Matayoshi Shinko, who learned the techniques on Tsuken-jima. It has also been suggested by Kise Fusei Hanshi, the founder of Kenshinkan and a prominent inheritor of Hohan Soken's Matsumura Seito Shorin Ryu, that the Matayoshi version originated with the Akamine family system on the island, positioning the kata within a long, family-based transmission that may stretch back for centuries.

Because of its oral tradition and household origins, accurately dating the kata is challenging. However, if the Akamine family system is indeed the source, its roots could extend back two to three hundred years. The sequence likely became recognizable as a formal kata in the late 18th or early 19th century, during the Satsuma's de facto control of the Ryukyus. At this time, the bo, a repurposed maritime tool, remained both practical and socially acceptable, which fostered the refinement of staff techniques for self-defense and communal safety.

Technically and culturally, Tsuken no Kun is a brilliant example of place-based innovation. Its emphasis on rapid directional shifts, tight angular entries, and strategic use of terrain and reach all point to the demands of island life. While broader Okinawan weapons traditions show some Chinese influence from maritime contact and trade, the structure and tactics of this kata are distinctly indigenous; a unique adaptation shaped by local needs rather than a direct transplant.

Applying Tsuken no Kun's Combat Wisdom

The kata Tsuken no Kun showcases a blend of rooted stability and fluid, deceptive motion. Its core principles emphasize practical combat needs, particularly in confined or unpredictable spaces. The stances within the kata are essential to this approach, combining deep, rooted postures with lighter, more mobile footwork. Movements often incorporate a firm base alongside fluid pivots, allowing for the rapid redirection of the bo.

The techniques and their applications are highly practical. Sweeping strikes designed to deflect an opponent's weapon and create openings for follow-up attacks are fundamental. Thrusts and pokes, utilizing the bo's full reach, create linear attacks aimed at the opponent's midline and face, while circular deflections are used to redirect incoming strikes with minimal effort, keeping the practitioner poised for a quick counterattack. These techniques are often linked in combination sequences, such as block-thrust-strike patterns, which prepare the practitioner to respond effectively to multi-directional threats.

The Matayoshi approach to Tsuken no Kun emphasizes an internal principle known as muchimi, which refers to a "sticky," heavy quality of movement. This principle ensures that the bo moves as a direct extension of the body, allowing for precise control and power. Breathing is carefully aligned with each strike to develop focused intent and deliver maximum force at the moment of impact. Together, these elements create a comprehensive system that enhances both offensive and defensive capabilities.

Tsuken no Kun's Evolving Traditions

The transmission of Tsuken no Kun is a characteristic feature of Okinawan kobudō, rooted in local practices and preserved through family lines. It was later systematized by itinerant teachers. Oral histories from Tsuken-jima attribute the core techniques of Tsuken no Kun to island bo specialists. These local instructors taught visiting martial artists, and it is believed that during these exchanges, Shinko Matayoshi learned the form. His son, Shinpo Matayoshi, then played a crucial role in formalizing Tsuken no Kun within the organized curriculum of Matayoshi Kobudō, helping to transmit the kata throughout Okinawa and to international students in the 20th century. Popular accounts suggest that the islanders of Tsuken used the kata's techniques to fend off pirates or settle disputes at the docks. While these tales blend verifiable local practices with folklore, they emphasize the kata's practical maritime origins. Because early transmissions were primarily private and oral, variations naturally developed as different teachers adapted the material to their specific needs and audiences. Figures like Kise Fusei and others have cited the Akamine family connection as one of several threads that contributed to later versions of the kata.

The Matayoshi interpretation emphasizes continuous flow and mobility, characterized by an embusen (performance line) and rhythm that favor smooth transitions and pivot-based redirection. In contrast, versions preserved or influenced by other prominent teachers, such as those associated with Taira, exhibit altered sequencing, tempo, and a stronger focus on segmented, heavy power generation. These differences reflect different pedagogical priorities: Matayoshi's approach highlights adaptability and fluidity, while other traditions tend to emphasize impact and specific technical markers.

The influence of Tsuken no Kun extends beyond its own practice. Elements such as pivot-driven redirection and compact, boat-friendly footwork reappear in later Matayoshi bo kata and contribute to the overall aesthetic of Matayoshi Kobudō. This results in a characteristic blend of flowing connection and practical application. Thus, the kata serves both as a preserved island repertoire and as a significant influence on subsequent staff training taught throughout Okinawa and beyond.

Tsuken no Kun's Lasting Impact

Rooted in the maritime life of Tsuken Island, Tsuken no Kun distills the practical combat needs and communal identity of a small seafaring community into a compact bojutsu system. The characteristics of the form, pivot-based redirection, tight angular entries, continuous flow, and whole-body integration, reflect techniques developed for the constraints of shipboard environments, docks, and narrow village streets. This kata has been preserved and systematized most visibly through the Matayoshi lineage, with links to local families such as the Akamines. It exemplifies Okinawan adaptability, combining economy of motion with effective mechanics.

Today, Tsuken no Kun serves both as a technical foundation for Matayoshi bo practice and as a living cultural link to Okinawa's coastal traditions. Each performance honors the island's legacy, transforming an everyday tool into a means of survival, while also transmitting important values such as adaptability, timing, and respect for lineage. Taught worldwide, the kata continues to shape staff work and preserve the memory of the fishermen-warriors and local teachers who created and safeguarded it, ensuring that a piece of Tsuken's history remains embodied in contemporary practice.

CHI'KIN BO
Okinawa's Mysterious Bo Tradition

Introduction to Chi'kin Bo

On a quiet day in the villages of the Ryukyu kingdom, including places like Nishihara, one might have once heard the rhythmic thunk of a bo striking the earth and the sharp whistle of wood cutting through the air. These sounds were not just exercise; they represented the language of a teacher who integrated samurai-influenced martial culture into Okinawan kobudō. Known in oral tradition as Chikin Kraka or Tsuken Mantaka, he is the figure behind a staff form that continues to echo his name in every thrust and sweep.

Preserved in the Matsumura Seito tradition as Chi'kin Bo, this kata is more than a simple sequence; it serves as a compact map of strategy, a living tribute to a warrior-teacher, and an example of how local practices can influence successive generations. This chapter traces the kata's journey, examining its probable origins, unpacking its technical elements such as pivots, angled entries, and footwork suitable for boat navigation, and following its transmission as teachers took on the responsibility of keeping the form alive. In doing so, we treat Chi'kin Bo not only as a practical bojutsu curriculum but also as an embodied fragment of Okinawa's rich martial history.

Unveiling Chi'kin Bo's Essence

- **Traditional Notation:** 津堅棒 or カナ書き「チキンボー」 (Okinawan reading for Tsuken Bō).
- **Script Breakdown:**
  - 津堅 "Tsuken/Chikin";
  - の posessive;
  - 棒 "staff."
- **Core Meaning:** "Tsuken staff," using the Okinawan pronunciation.
- **Modern Interpretations:** Used to distinguish dialectal lineage.
- **Conflicting Ideas & Origins:** Sometimes treated as a specific variant; sometimes as a synonym of Tsuken no Kun.

Chi'kin Bo, also known as Chikin no Kun or, in standard Japanese, Tsuken no Kun, carries both geographic and personal significance. The most literal translation of its name, 津堅の棍, reads in Japanese as Tsuken no Kun, meaning "the bo of Tsuken." The final character may appear as 棍 (kun) or 棒 (bo) in different sources; both terms refer to a long wooden staff and are used interchangeably in kobudō naming.

Importantly, "Chi'kin" is not a different word but rather the pronunciation of the same name in the Okinawan dialect (Uchina-guchi). While mainland Japanese renders the island name as "Tsuken," it is pronounced locally as "Chi'kin." This dialectal difference accounts for the various spellings; Chi'kin, Chikin, and Tsuken; found in oral accounts and Romanized texts. Oral tradition connects this form to an individual known as Chikin Kraka or Tsuken Mantaka. The personal name and the place name thus overlap, allowing the kata's title to legitimately reference both a locality and a teacher.

This dual reference reflects common practice in Okinawa, where kata names often signify a place, person, or local style. For Okinawan practitioners, the name serves as a compact claim of origin and authenticity, evoking Tsuken's maritime environment and/or the lineage of a named master. However, it is important to note that the geographic-personal label should not be interpreted as evidence of a single, unchanging technique. Like many place-named kata, Chi'kin Bo has diversified among different schools, even while the name preserves a shared origin story and cultural identity.

Chi'kin Bo's Historical Roots

The recognized origin of Chi'kin Bo is rooted in the life and practices of the teacher known in oral tradition as Chikin Kraka or Tsuken Mantaka. His home in Nishihara village served as a training ground for the techniques that eventually coalesced into the kata. Local accounts suggest that he had a samurai-influenced background, whether through lineage, service, or martial association, which helped shape the disciplined and combative nature of the form.

Historians place Mantaka's active period in the mid-to-late 19th century, a time when Okinawan martial arts were taught privately due to the social pressures imposed by Satsuma's control. Contemporary accounts record Mantaka training with notable figures such as Tomigusuku Seiko no Ueekata and possibly the earlier teacher Bushi Sakiyama Kitoku. Some versions of the story also suggest that he may have traveled to or been influenced by the Yaeyama Islands, which could have introduced additional regional bojutsu techniques into his repertoire. These connections are primarily conveyed through lineage testimony rather than formal documentation, which is typical for Okinawan weapon arts of that era.

The social context explains why the bo became Mantaka's primary focus. A long staff, readily available as a boat pole or farming implement, remained a practical and socially acceptable tool when formal weapons were restricted. Therefore, Chi'kin Bo reflects functionality born out of necessity, featuring compact and efficient techniques suitable for confined spaces such as decks and docks, as well as methods for defending against both armed and unarmed opponents. The kata was designed to train whole-body control, balance, timing, and the effective use of the staff's full length.

Technically, the form is grounded in Okinawan staff practice but exhibits signs of broader influences. Maritime trade and cultural exchange suggest that certain movements may have been derived from Chinese staff methods, while principles from spear fighting contribute to its flowing yet forceful rhythm, indicating both local adaptation and external influences.

Applying Chi'kin Bo's Combat Wisdom

Chi'kin Bo, in Hohan Soken's Matsumura Seito tradition, emphasizes stability combined with nimble evasion. The practice focuses on rooted stances for structural support, engaging the hips and aligning the spine, while the footwork highlights precise control over distance. This includes stepping off-line to evade incoming strikes and then closing in or angling to counterattack. Key elements such as ma-ai (fighting distance), timing, and hip connection are prioritized, ensuring that every strike or thrust is supported by the body's center rather than relying solely on arm reach.

The kata is organized around a small, repeated set of tactical techniques. It employs sweeping parries using circular, efficient motions of the bo to deflect and redirect attacks, rather than confronting them head-on. Low sweeps and targeted foot attacks are designed to unbalance an opponent and create openings, while extended thrusts utilize the staff's reach to keep an adversary at bay. The transitions within the sequence are intentionally ambiguous, allowing many movements to serve dual purposes as both defense and preparation for an immediate counterattack, thereby disguising intent and conserving momentum.

The kata also features a distinctive practical repertoire in its bunkai, including techniques for intercepting and neutralizing cuts from bladed weapons, trapping or binding an opponent's staff, and converting that control into disarming or finishing techniques. Close-range responses such as short upward strikes to the ribs or throat, rapid cross-body blocks leading into counters, and quick pivots that change the line of attack translate the kata into realistic self-defense scenarios. Traditional anecdotal tactics, preserved through oral teachings, like quick sand scoops or sand throws to distract an opponent during coastal encounters, reflect the island context in which some practical methods were developed.

Stylistically, the kata balances linear power with circular mobility. Spiral or torque mechanics are employed in certain thrusts to enhance penetration while stabilizing the body. Pivot-based redirection is a hallmark of this form, allowing practitioners to capitalize on an opponent's momentum. Adapted for confined maritime environments such as decks, docks, and narrow lanes, the movements are compact and efficient, prioritizing safe recovery and rapid re-engagement over large, telegraphed motions.

Training in the kata with a focus on hip connection, weight distribution, and transitional timing reveals these applications clearly. Partner drills that emphasize binding, trapping, and thrust timing, along with solo repetition of the embusen and rhythm, help students internalize how sweeping parries can turn into offensive opportunities and how the bo's length can be utilized to control space and deliver decisive strikes.

Chi'kin Bo's Evolving Traditions

The transmission of Chi'kin Bo follows the familiar Okinawan pattern of private teaching, family connections, and eventual systematization by influential teachers. The oral tradition attributes the origins of the kata to Chikin Kraka (Tsuken Mantaka), a bojutsu specialist from Nishihara. He trained under Tomigusuku Seiko no Ueekata and, by some accounts, studied with Bushi Sakiyama Kitoku, a figure believed to have ties to Ryu Ryu Ko and Ason in China. These personal connections help explain the kata's blend of practical Okinawan techniques with elements derived from broader regional staff and spear practices.

Mantaka entrusted the kata to a local custodian, Bushi Komesu no Tanme (Komesu Ushi), who in turn passed it on to Hohan Soken. Soken's adoption of the kata was pivotal; he incorporated Chi'kin Bo into the Matsumura-Seito curriculum, thereby framing it within his comprehensive teaching program that linked karate and kobudō. Recognizing the importance of continuity and adaptability, Soken appointed Kise Fusei as his successor. Kise went on to establish the Kenshinkan and carry Chi'kin Bo into the Okinawan Matsumura Seito Karate and Kobudō Federation, ensuring the kata's organized transmission into the modern era and beyond Okinawa's shores.

Variation naturally emerged from these developments. The Kenshinkan version of Chi'kin Bo remains closely aligned with Soken's teaching methods, emphasizing flow, timing, and the specific embusen preserved within that lineage. In contrast, other branches that trace back to Mantaka exhibit alternative rhythms, tempos, and minor sequence differences. These divergences reflect typical factors in Okinawan transmission, including individual body types, teaching priorities (such as power versus fluidity), training environments (village docks versus dojos), and the pedagogical needs of successive students.

Chi'kin Bo's influence is evident within the Kenshinkan repertoire itself: long-range thrusting mechanics, pivot-based evasions, and compact transition movements are recurrent in later bo kata and inform the overall staff methodology of the school. In this way, the kata serves both as a preserved island art and as a foundational source for subsequent kobudō traditions.

Chi'kin Bo's Lasting Impact

Chi'kin Bo serves as a direct, embodied link to the 19th-century bojutsu practitioner known as Chikin Kraka (Tsuken Mantaka). Through a lineage that includes figures such as Komesu, Hohan Soken, and the Kise line, the kata has preserved a practical fighting mindset characterized by compact, ship-and-shore friendly techniques. These techniques train balance, timing, and effective use of reach. This historical lineage anchors the form while allowing for minor variations that naturally arise from personal transmission and differing teaching priorities.

Within the Kenshinkan and related Matsumura-Seito circles, Chi'kin Bo is not merely a museum piece; it is a living tradition. It is actively taught, practiced, and adapted for contemporary students as both technical bojutsu and a cultural memory. Each training session preserves tactical lessons and reflects the island-born aesthetics that have shaped them. Under the guidance of Kise Isao, until his passing in February 2025, the kata's influence expanded internationally, ensuring that the rhythm and principles of Nishihara's staff fighting continue to resonate in dojos around the world.

The enduring value of the kata lies in its dual role as both a practical method and a repository of lineage. As teachers and students keep Chi'kin Bo in active practice, they preserve an element of Okinawan maritime culture, maintain a tested set of staff tactics useful in various contexts, and honor the lineage that has transmitted the form from a village training ground to the global martial arts community.

CHATAN YARA NO KUN

Okinawa's Legendary Hero Staff

Introduction to Chatan Yara no Kun

The name Chatan Yara no Kun carries both historical and legendary significance, conjuring images of the bo-wielding warriors of old Okinawa. More than a mere sequence of staff maneuvers, this kata serves as a living record of the island's martial heritage. It is attributed to Yara of Chatan, a pivotal figure whose life bridges the gap between documented history and oral tradition. The kata exemplifies the fusion of indigenous Ryukyuan fighting styles with Chinese martial arts, which were introduced through Okinawa's vibrant trade and cultural exchange networks.

Throughout generations, Chatan Yara no Kun has preserved not only practical combat principles but also insights into the era when Okinawan martial arts evolved through both necessity and diplomacy. Its techniques demonstrate the strategic use of distance, timing, and adaptability; hallmarks of Okinawan kobudō. In this chapter, we will explore the kata's origins and its connection to Chatan Yara himself, analyze its technical and tactical features, trace its journey through various lineages, and consider its lasting relevance in the modern martial arts world.

Exploring the Essence of Chatan Yara no Kun

- **Traditional Notation:** 北谷屋良の棍 (Chatan Yara no Kon).
- **Script Breakdown:**
  - 北谷屋良 "Chatan Yara" (person); literally "Yara of Chatan"
  - の posessive;
  - 棒 "staff."
- **Core Meaning:** "Chatan Yara's staff."
- **Modern Interpretations:** Found across Tomari-influenced kobudō.
- **Conflicting Ideas & Origins:** Minor divergences among Shitō/Matayoshi/Ryūkyū groups.

The kata's name, Chatan Yara no Kun (北谷屋良の棍), translates to "The Staff of Yara from Chatan." Its written form combines kanji and katakana, a practice commonly found in Okinawan martial arts that reflects both its local origins and its integration into broader Japanese writing systems.

The name directly connects the kata to Yara of Chatan, a legendary figure traditionally credited with either creating or transmitting various forms. Like many Okinawan kata, its exact authorship is challenging to verify, and some historians suggest that while Yara may have codified or popularized the kata, its techniques likely drew on multiple influences over generations; a practice typical of Okinawa's dynamic martial exchange with China and other regional traditions.

Beyond the technical attribution, the name holds deep cultural significance. Okinawan kata are often named after notable individuals, not just as an acknowledgment of authorship but as a tribute to the teacher's legacy and community roots. In this regard, Chatan Yara no Kun serves as both a historical marker and a symbol of Okinawa's martial identity. It preserves the memory of Yara's role in the dissemination of staff techniques while situating the kata within the broader context of Ryukyuan cultural heritage.

Chatan Yara no Kun's Historical Roots

Chatan Yara no Kun traces its lineage to one of Okinawa's most revered martial figures, a man named Yara (1668–1746), who was a native of Chatan village in central Okinawa. Born into the educated yukatchu class, Yara is recognized as a pioneer of Okinawan te and kobudō, living during a time that blurs the line between historical fact and legend.

Accounts agree that during his youth, Yara traveled to China, most likely to Fujian, where he spent nearly two decades studying martial arts under renowned teachers such as Wong Chung-Yoh. He trained in both unarmed combat, including various forms of Chinese quanfa, and classical weapon systems, experiences that profoundly influenced his later teachings.

Upon his return in the late 17th century, Okinawa was under Satsuma domain, a period characterized by cultural blending and the discreet preservation of martial practices. Yara became a key figure in this synthesis, adapting Chinese methods to local contexts and emphasizing practical, combative application over mere display. His influence is seen in multiple kata attributed to him, including Chatan Yara no Kun, Chatan Yara no Sai, and a version of Kushanku. Through disciples such as Takahara Peichin, Yara's teachings spread widely, helping to shape the technical and philosophical foundations of Okinawan martial arts. One notable anecdote involves Yara's encounter with a Satsuma samurai. According to legend, Yara disarmed and killed the samurai using an oar (eku), showcasing his exceptional martial prowess.

The creation of Chatan Yara no Kun likely served both practical and cultural purposes: it was a means to codify staff techniques for self-defense and a way to preserve martial heritage. The kata's movements reflect a fusion of indigenous Okinawan tactics with Chinese principles, making it a bridge between these two traditions. As such, Chatan Yara no Kun stands as a testament to the dynamic flow of martial knowledge across borders and generations, embodying the very process that gave rise to Okinawa's unique and enduring martial culture.

Applying Chatan Yara no Kun's Combat Wisdom

Chatan Yara no Kun captures the essence of Okinawan staff work through a seamless integration of balance, power, and tactical adaptability. This kata trains practitioners to effectively wield the full length of the bo, allowing for smooth transitions between long-range thrusts, mid-range sweeps, and close-quarters defenses. Its techniques encompass a versatile range of thrusts, downward and diagonal cuts, and dynamic sweeping motions. These are complemented by defensive maneuvers, such as rising and double blocks, which highlight the staff's dual offensive and protective potential.

Beyond simply being a list of strikes, the form teaches essential principles of effective bojutsu: stable stances that provide support without compromising mobility, coordinated breathing that aligns timing and power, and the cultivation of focused intent with every movement. Through its flowing transitions and controlled rhythms, Chatan Yara no Kun embodies the broader principles of Okinawan martial arts, where fluidity and precision come together with practical application. By exploring its bunkai, practitioners not only enhance their technical skills but also gain insights into the kata's historical and cultural significance as a living tradition of both self-defense and artistic expression.

Chatan Yara no Kun's Evolving Traditions

The transmission of Chatan Yara no Kun illustrates both the resilience of Okinawan martial traditions and the creative interpretations of successive generations. Yara's teachings were initially passed on to his student, Takahara Peichin, who played a crucial role in spreading the form. Takahara's instruction significantly influenced Sakugawa Kangi, whose later prominence in the development of Okinawan karate helped elevate the visibility of Yara's methods. Through these early connections, the kata became embedded in multiple lineages, preserving its core principles while allowing for stylistic variations.

Over time, Chatan Yara no Kun has evolved differently across various schools of kobudō. The Kyan lineage emphasizes smooth, flowing transitions, fluidity, and natural posture, reflecting Chotoku Kyan's personal style and focus on adaptable, practical defense. In contrast, the Matsubayashi-Ryu lineage prioritizes simplicity and directness, highlighting rooted stances and strong foundational techniques for maximum practical application. The Taira/Inoue lineage presents a more asymmetrical and technically demanding version, showcasing its complexity through sparse repetition and challenging sequences.

These variations do not detract from the kata's essence; instead, they demonstrate how different interpretations, teaching approaches, and tactical priorities shape its expression. Comparing the versions across different lineages provides insight into Okinawa's diverse kobudō traditions and the enduring adaptability of its martial arts.

Chatan Yara no Kun's Lasting Impact

Chatan Yara no Kun is a testament to the depth and resilience of Okinawan martial arts. Rooted in the teachings of the legendary Yara of Chatan, whose extensive studies in China influenced the techniques and philosophy of Okinawan fighting, this kata embodies a sophisticated blend of offense, defense, and adaptability. Its movements develop balance, generate power, and demonstrate practical application, reflecting a tradition that values both effectiveness and artistry.

Passed down through generations, from Takahara Peichin to Sakugawa Kangi and beyond, the kata has evolved within multiple lineages. Each lineage has preserved its core principles while adding unique stylistic nuances. Its lasting presence across different schools not only highlights its technical richness but also its cultural significance as a bridge between historical heritage and contemporary practice.

For practitioners, engaging with Chatan Yara no Kun is more than just mastering a series of staff techniques; it is a way to connect with a living tradition. By studying this kata, martial artists link themselves to centuries of Okinawan martial history, sustaining the legacy of Yara's teachings and ensuring the vitality of the island's unique martial heritage for future generations.

Matsu Higa no Kun
Okinawa's Resolute Staff Mastery

Introduction to Matsu Higa no Kun

Imagine a bo kata so fluid and precise that each strike and block feels like a conversation with the warrior past of Okinawa. Matsu Higa no Kun, named after the semi-legendary Pechin Matsu Higa, stands as a testament to the bushi class of the Ryukyu Kingdom. This form blends practical combat techniques with the cultural ethos of a kingdom under pressure. Rooted in the late 19th century, this classical kobudō form showcases the versatility of the bo through swift thrusts, sweeping blocks, and seamless transitions that reflect real-world defense against armed opponents. Attributed to Matsu Higa Pechin, a martial artist from Hamahiga Island who also codified the sai and tonfa kata, this form draws influences from Chinese quan fa and Okinawan ingenuity, adapted to the weapon bans of the Satsuma era. It has been preserved in lineages such as Ryukyu Kobudō Hozon Shinkokai and Matayoshi Kobudō, complementing karate forms like Gojushiho and embodying the disciplined resilience of the Yukatchu. This chapter explores its origins, technical depth, and enduring significance, revealing how Matsu Higa no Kun intertwines history, identity, and martial artistry into a living legacy of Okinawan kobudō.

Exploring the Essence of Matsu Higa no Kun

•**Traditional Notation:** 松比嘉の棒, romanized variously as Matsu Higa, Matsu Higa no Tanmei, or Matsuhiga.

•**Script Breakdown:**

　　○松比嘉 romanized variously as "Matsu Higa," or" Matsuhiga"

　　○の posessive;

　　○棒 "staff."

•**Core Meaning:** "Matsuhiga's staff."

•**Modern Interpretations:** Most modern historians treat him as a real but semi-legendary instructor, preserved mainly through weapon kata attribution..

•**Conflicting Ideas & Origins:** Name/reading confusion ("Matsuhiga" vs. "Matsu Higa") persists in English-language materials.

The name Matsu Higa no Kun (松比嘉の棍) is an integral part of Okinawa's martial arts history, linking a person, place, and weapon. Matsu Higa (松比嘉) refers to a semi-legendary pechin from Hamahiga Island, a small but culturally rich island off Okinawa's east coast, that is associated with Ryukyuan creation myths. The particle no (の) connects this figure to Kun (棍), which refers to the six-foot hardwood bo that is central to the kata, translating to "The Staff of Matsu Higa." This kanji-based naming combines Okinawan and Japanese traditions, grounding the kata in both regional identity and the practical artistry of kobudō.

There is some historical debate regarding the figure of Matsu Higa. Most sources point to a 19th-century martial artist (1790–1870), a pechin who codified various kata for the sai, tonfa, and bo, including this one, under the influence of Chinese quan fa. However, some oral traditions merge him with an earlier Hama Higa Pechin (1663–1738), who was known for demonstrating sai-jutsu before Japan's 5th Tokugawa Shogun. The timeline suggests that they were two distinct individuals, but later narratives conflated their legacies due to their shared island heritage. Regardless, the name honors the pechin class's role in preserving martial knowledge during the Satsuma weapon bans, embodying duty and resilience.

Matsu Higa no Kun represents more than just a name; it signifies a legacy. Preserved in lineages such as Ryukyu Kobudō and Matayoshi Kobudō, it connects the bo, a practical weapon and cultural emblem, to Hamahiga's heritage. This reflects Okinawa's complex blend of memory, identity, and martial tradition.

Matsu Higa no Kun's Historical Roots

For many, Matsu Higa no Kun is a fundamental aspect of Okinawan kobudō, with its roots tracing back to the declining years of the Ryukyu Kingdom. It embodies the resilience of a warrior culture under duress. This bo kata is attributed to Matsu Higa Pechin (circa 1790–1870), a compact yet formidable pechin from Hamahiga Island. His kata reflects the disciplined ethos of Okinawa's aristocratic bushi class. Oral traditions depict him as a martial titan, standing just over five feet tall but powerful enough to crush coconuts by hand and fend off pirates. This blend of myth and practical skills highlights his role as a royal guard. His codification of bo, sai, and tonfa kata, including this one, influenced prominent figures like Takahara Peichin and Sakugawa Kanga, solidifying his legacy within the Shorin-ryu and kobudō lineages.

Confusion sometimes arises due to an earlier figure, Hama Higa Pechin (1663–1738), who was known for demonstrating saijutsu before Japan's fifth Tokugawa Shogun. Although their shared island origins contribute to this mix-up, scholars consistently link Matsu Higa no Kun to the 19th century, corresponding with the later figure's era of martial systematization. Following the Satsuma rule after 1609, which limited weapons, pechin like Matsu Higa had to adapt tools such as the bo for defense and law enforcement. He drew inspiration from Chinese quan fa and indigenous Okinawan techniques to create a kata that balances fluid strikes and blocks with practical combat applications, ensuring its effectiveness and ease of transmission.

Matsu Higa's codification was both a necessity and a legacy: it was a response to political constraints and a commitment to preserving Ryukyuan martial heritage. This kata is preserved in lineages like the Ryukyu Kobudō Hozon Shinkokai and Matayoshi Kobudō. Matsu Higa no Kun stands as a testament to Okinawa's ability to adapt and thrive, weaving local duty with global influences into a timeless expression of martial artistry.

Applying Matsu Higa no Kun's Combat Wisdom

Matsu Higa no Kun is a prime example of bo-jutsu in Okinawan kobudō, blending the practicality of the Pechin warrior with the versatile power of the staff. Rooted in the martial ethos of the Ryukyu Kingdom, this kata employs stances such as zenkutsu dachi, kiba dachi, and hachiji dachi to establish balance and maximize force. These stances flow seamlessly, reflecting Matsu Higa's emphasis on efficiency and fluid transitions, allowing practitioners to shift effortlessly between offense and defense in real-world scenarios.

The techniques within this kata showcase the adaptability of the bo, featuring overhead strikes, precise thrusts, and sweeping blocks. These techniques can be executed with both centered grips for control and full-length swings for greater reach. A unique aspect of this form is the incorporation of sand-flicking movements, which likely aim to disorient opponents, along with multi-level blocks that blend defense into attack. The bunkai of these movements demonstrate their utility in disarming armed opponents or countering multiple attackers, reflecting the Pechin's duty to maintain order even under weapon bans.

Core principles such as controlled breathing, intense focus, and grounded stability elevate the kata beyond mere technique, fostering internal discipline and combat readiness. Preserved in lineages like Ryukyu Kobudō and Matayoshi Kobudō, Matsu Higa no Kun embodies the bushi's balance of strength, strategy, and cultural resilience, making it a vital link to Okinawa's martial heritage.

Matsu Higa no Kun's Evolving Traditions

A fundamental aspect of Okinawan kobudō, Matsu Higa no Kun has developed through various lineages, each preserving the essence of the kata while adding unique elements. Originating with Matsu Higa Pechin, this kata was passed down through disciples and has influenced modern systems such as Ryukyu Kobujutsu and Matayoshi Kobudō. These lineages showcase variations shaped by regional influences, teaching methods, and the interpretations of different masters, reflecting Okinawa's dynamic martial heritage.

In the Ryukyu Kobujutsu lineage, codified by Taira Shinken, the kata emphasizes efficient and dynamic movements. It features sweeping circular bo motions performed behind the back, powerful strikes delivered from kiba dachi or zenkutsu dachi, and the distinctive sand-flicking technique designed to disorient opponents. Taira's system, focused on documenting Okinawan weapon arts, prioritizes the full length and momentum of the bo for practical combat training. In contrast, the Matayoshi Kobudō lineage, taught by Matayoshi Shinko and Shinpo, emphasizes comprehensive bunkai. Its version of the kata highlights nuanced hip rotation and fluid stance transitions, tailoring movements to specific self-defense scenarios and making subtle adjustments in body mechanics to maximize power.

These variations arise from regional practices, individual teaching styles, and the holistic approach of Okinawan training, where masters often blended techniques from different weapons. The kata's influence also extends to other bo forms, enriching kobudō curricula. However, tracing these exact impacts can be challenging due to oral traditions and secretive transmissions. Distinct from other bo lineages like Chinen or Soeishi, Matsu Higa no Kun remains a vibrant testament to Okinawa's adaptable martial legacy, balancing tradition with innovation.

Matsu Higa no Kun's Lasting Impact

Matsu Higa no Kun is an important aspect of Okinawan kobudō, representing the legacy of Matsu Higa Pechin and the resilient spirit of the warrior class of the Ryukyu Kingdom. Rooted in the cultural heritage of Hamahiga Island, this bo kata showcases the Pechin's disciplined efficiency. It combines influences from Chinese quan fa with the practicality of Okinawan martial arts, resulting in fluid strikes, blocks, and sand-flicking techniques suitable for real-world combat.

Passed down through various Kobudō masters, Matsu Higa no Kun has evolved across different lineages. Notable styles include the dynamic circular movements of Ryukyu Kobujutsu under Taira Shinken and the precise, application-focused approach of Matayoshi Kobudō. Each variation adds to its depth and complexity.

Today, Matsu Higa no Kun is preserved within multiple systems and remains a cornerstone of kobudō, embodying the martial ethos and cultural pride of the bushi. As practitioners practice the bo, they connect with centuries of history, linking past struggles under Satsuma rule to modern dojos. This kata is more than just a sequence of movements; it serves as a living connection to Okinawa's rich martial heritage, promoting values of adaptability, strength, and tradition for future generations.

SECTION II – SAIJ-UTSU KATA

Okinawa's Trident: The Iron Fork of Defense

The sai is a short, trident-shaped iron weapon known for its unique defensive capabilities. While it is often associated with Japanese police tools, in Okinawa, it has been adapted for both civil defense and martial arts training. Its origins may trace back to Southeast Asian and Chinese weapons. Still, Okinawan tradition firmly establishes it within the Ryukyuan martial repertoire during the kingdom's maritime trade era.

The sai is particularly effective for trapping, parrying, and disarming opponents wielding weapons such as swords or staffs. It can also deliver thrusts and blunt strikes. In Okinawan culture, the sai symbolizes order and control; it is a weapon that neutralizes an opponent's advantage while embodying the disciplined, defensive spirit of martial arts. Its significance in kata demonstrates the Ryukyuan ability to combine practicality with cultural symbolism.

CHATAN YARA NO SAI
Okinawa's Iron Shield

Introduction to Chatan Yara no Sai

Few kata capture the ingenuity of Okinawan kobudō quite like Chatan Yara no Sai. Performed with twin truncheon-like weapons, this kata combines elegant spins with sharp, decisive thrusts and traps, transforming simple iron tools into extensions of both defense and offense. To the uninitiated, its techniques may appear theatrical, but behind the flashy arcs and sudden snaps lies a record of practical combat methods, offering a glimpse into the cultural fabric of Okinawa.

Traditionally, the form is attributed to Chatan Yara, an 18th-century figure renowned not only for his skill with weapons but also for his role in shaping Okinawan martial culture during a period of significant Chinese influence. Accounts suggest that Yara trained in China before returning to Okinawa, where he transmitted a blend of empty-hand and weapons techniques to a select circle of disciples. The sai kata that bears his name reflects this synthesis, featuring fast and precise manipulation, sudden changes of rhythm, and the ability to trap, strike, and counter with seamless efficiency.

This chapter explores Chatan Yara no Sai as both a historical artifact and a living practice. We will examine its roots and the question of its attribution to Yara, situate it within broader kobudō transmission lines, and analyze its technical and cultural essence. Additionally, we will consider how the kata has been preserved, interpreted, and adapted in modern dojos, demonstrating how a weapon once wielded on Okinawa's streets still embodies timeless principles of strategy, control, and discipline.

Exploring the Essence of Chatan Yara no Sai

- **Traditional Notation:** 北谷屋良の釵.
- **Script Breakdown:**
  - 北谷屋良 "Chatan Yara" (person); literally "Yara of Chatan"
  - の possessive;
  - 釵 "sai."
- **Core Meaning:** "Chatan Yara's sai."
- **Modern Interpretations:** Often paired with his bō curriculum.
- **Conflicting Ideas & Origins:** Stable name and etymology.

The name "Chatan Yara no Sai" carries multiple layers of meaning that reflect Okinawan history and martial tradition. "Chatan" refers to the coastal region of Okinawa from which Yara originated, situating this form within a specific cultural and geographic context. "Yara" identifies the legendary martial artist himself, who is remembered in both oral tradition and fragmentary records as a skilled fighter, both armed and unarmed. Finally, "Sai" (釵) designates the weapon central to the kata; the iron truncheon with its distinctive prongs, once used in Okinawa for defense, control, and countering armed opponents. Together, these elements mark the form as both a technical curriculum and a tribute to the individual and place that shaped it.

Unlike some kata that are written in katakana to preserve their Chinese phonetics, "Chatan Yara no Sai" is written in kanji. This underscores its long-standing integration into Okinawan martial practice rather than highlighting external influences. While the meaning of the characters is straightforward, the figure of Yara himself is more elusive. Some historians view him as a semi-legendary figure whose deeds blend with folktale, while others suggest plausible connections to later teachers. In this way, the kata embodies both the functional training of kobudō and the cultural mythology that gives these forms their significance.

Naming the kata after Yara reflects a broader Okinawan custom of honoring teachers and local heroes by naming martial forms after them. Therefore, practicing "Chatan Yara no Sai" is more than just learning a sequence of movements; it is a means of preserving memory, connecting today's practitioners with the stories of Okinawa's past, and carrying forward the legacy of one of its most iconic martial figures.

Chatan Yara no Sai's Historical Roots

The story of Chatan Yara no Sai begins with Chatan Yara, a figure remembered in oral tradition as both a skilled martial artist and a community leader from the Chatan region of Okinawa. Accounts describe him as a warrior-scholar of the ueekata class who traveled to China, where he is said to have studied various empty-hand methods and weapons before returning to Okinawa. Upon his return, Yara gained a reputation as a teacher and protector, credited with spreading the use of the sai, bo, and other weapons across the island. He is not only associated with the sai kata but also with Chatan Yara no Kon, suggesting that his influence extended into multiple aspects of Okinawan kobudō.

Most sources trace the kata's origins to the 18th century, during the Satsuma occupation, a time when official restrictions on weapon ownership prompted Okinawans to preserve their martial arts discreetly. The sai, in particular, held a significant role in Okinawan society, serving both as a practical tool for defense and as an emblem of law enforcement, carried by officials known as chikusaji. Its possible roots may lie elsewhere, drawing inspiration from Chinese truncheons or Indian weapons; however, in Okinawa, the sai developed a uniquely local identity tied to both civilian defense and authority.

The kata itself likely served a dual purpose. On one hand, it was pragmatic, training practitioners in the use of sai against bladed weapons and staffs with techniques that emphasize trapping, deflecting, and counter-striking. On the other hand, it functioned as a vehicle for cultural memory, preserving the legacy of Chatan Yara and infusing elements of Chinese-inspired fluidity within the sharp, linear framework of Okinawan Shorin-based stances. Its survival into modern times is primarily due to preservationists like Taira Shinken, who cataloged and codified Okinawan kobudō kata in the 20th century, and later to teachers such as Matayoshi Shinpo, who ensured its inclusion in established kobudō curricula. Today, the form remains present in Matayoshi traditions, Shorin-ryu–derived schools, and systems like Kenshinkan, continuing to carry forward both its combative value and its role as a connection to Okinawa's martial past.

Applying Chatan Yara no Sai's Combat Wisdom

At the heart of Chatan Yara no Sai lies a blend of fluidity and control, with every movement designed to showcase the unique strengths of the sai while reinforcing the foundational mechanics of Okinawan martial culture. The kata emphasizes rooted stances that provide both forward drive and lateral stability, ensuring the practitioner can close the distance with decisive speed or retreat while maintaining balance. These transitions reflect the Shorin-ryu focus on economy of motion, which is characterized by being swift, efficient, and adaptable.

One of the most significant features of the form is its demand for ambidextrous dexterity. Practitioners are required to shift the weapon smoothly from one grip to another, alternating offense and defense with equal proficiency in either hand. This ambidexterity mirrors the Shōrin approach to empty-hand kata, where agility and symmetry are key to mastering timing and distance.

The technical repertoire of the kata is both rich and varied. Direct thrusts (tsuki) form its striking core, aimed at vital targets such as the solar plexus, throat, or ribs. Blocks (uke) utilize the prongs (yoku) of the sai to intercept or deflect powerful strikes, particularly from the bō. The weapon's design also allows for more subtle tactics, such as hooking and trapping an opponent's staff or blade before controlling and countering decisively. Flipping motions, where the sai rotates between an "open" and "closed" grip, demonstrate the adaptability of the weapon, enabling rapid shifts between defensive deflections and sharp offensive thrusts.

Beyond the outward techniques, the kata also cultivates essential internal qualities. Proper breath control underpins the rhythm of execution, lending power to strikes while maintaining calm focus under pressure. The sai's solid weight requires strong wrist and forearm conditioning, reinforcing stability and precision over time. Additionally, the kata's balanced, often symmetrical sequences challenge the practitioner to develop mental focus and bodily awareness, which not only enhances technical skill but also fosters composure and confidence.

Through this combination of structure, adaptability, and inner refinement, Chatan Yara no Sai becomes more than just a set of techniques; it is a disciplined study of how Okinawan martial artists harness the unique potential of the sai to address the challenges of both combat and personal development.

Chatan Yara no Sai's Evolving Traditions

Like many Okinawan kata, Chatan Yara no Sai did not remain fixed in a single form; it evolved as it passed through different teachers and lineages. Its preservation owes much to Taira Shinken, whose efforts to codify and standardize Okinawan kobudō ensured the kata's survival and dissemination. From his work, it entered the Matayoshi system, where it became a central sai form, and from there, it spread into Shorin-ryu–based schools worldwide.

The variations that exist today reflect the philosophies of their respective traditions. The Matayoshi lineage emphasizes circularity and continuity, highlighting smooth transitions and flowing arcs of movement that echo Chinese-influenced body mechanics. In contrast, Shorin-ryu versions tend toward sharper lines and more abrupt transitions, embodying the school's preference for directness and rapid engagement.

These differences are not contradictions; rather, they demonstrate Okinawan adaptability. Masters tailored the form to their instructional goals, whether to highlight aesthetic flow for performance, sharpen technical precision for teaching, or emphasize combative realism for application. Such diversity reveals the living character of Okinawan martial arts, where kata are not static relics but dynamic vessels for transmitting core principles across generations.

The influence of Chatan Yara no Sai also extends beyond its practice. Along with forms like Hama Higa no Sai, it helped establish structured sai curricula within kobudō systems, ensuring that students encountered complementary approaches to the weapon. Additionally, stories of Yara wielding the sai to protect villagers from bandits imbued the kata with cultural resonance, linking its practice to Okinawan identity and communal memory.

In this way, Chatan Yara no Sai stands as both a technical tradition and a cultural symbol. Shaped by multiple lineages yet united in spirit, it reminds practitioners that Okinawan kobudō has always thrived on adaptation while maintaining a connection to its roots.

Chatan Yara no Sai's Lasting Impact

Key insights into Chatan Yara no Sai reveal its deep connections to Okinawan history and culture. The name itself links this kata practice to a legendary figure from Okinawa, underscoring its significance in martial traditions. Historically, Chatan Yara no Sai represents a unique blend of Chinese influence and Okinawan adaptation, particularly during the Satsuma occupation, which shaped its development.

From a technical perspective, this form emphasizes the cultivation of ambidexterity, wrist strength, and the management of distance, making it particularly effective for practical combat against armed opponents. Over time, the traditions surrounding Chatan Yara no Sai have branched out across various lineages, each preserving different facets of the form and ensuring that its rich legacy continues to thrive.

The form's enduring legacy is as one of the most widely practiced sai katas, linking modern kobudō practitioners with centuries of Okinawan martial history. It serves as a training tool, a cultural artifact, and a living tradition.

In conclusion, for today's martial artist, practicing Chatan Yara no Sai is not only an exercise in technique but also an act of preservation; a way to honor Chatan Yara's ingenuity and to ensure that Okinawa's weapon heritage continues to live on through the movements of each new generation.

HAMA HIGA NO SAI
Okinawa's Island Trident

Introduction to Hama Higa no Sai

Imagine a kata so intricately woven that each flick of the sai and rooted stance tells a compelling story, not just of combat, but of the enduring spirit of Okinawa. Hama Higa no Sai, named after the historic Hamahiga Island in the Yokatsu archipelago, is a valuable piece of kobudō that combines practical self-defense with the cultural legacy of the Ryukyu Kingdom. Its movements carry the weight of history, echoing the resilience of an island people who have navigated centuries of political upheaval.

Emerging in the late 17th century, this kata is associated with the legendary Hama Higa Pechin (1663–1738), a martial artist who is said to have demonstrated saijutsu before Japan's 5th Tokugawa Shogun, Tsunayoshi. Some oral traditions connect him with Matsu Higa, potentially a descendant, blending Chinese-influenced techniques with Okinawan ingenuity. The kata's dynamic blocks, precise thrusts, and rapidly shifting stances reflect the adaptability developed under Satsuma's weapon bans, embodying the warrior ethos of the bushi class.

Hama Higa no Sai has been preserved within several lineages, complementing karate forms while highlighting the distinct role of kobudō. This chapter delves into its origins, exploring its namesake island, historical roots, technical depth, and variations in lineage, attempting to distinguish myth from fact. By situating the kata within its socio-political context, we reveal its technical brilliance and symbolic significance in modern Okinawan martial arts.

Exploring the Essence of Hama Higa no Sai

- **Traditional Notation:** 浜比嘉の釵 (Hamahiga no Sai).
- **Script Breakdown:**
    - 浜比嘉 (Hamahiga island/family);
    - の posessive;
    - 釵 "sai."
- **Core Meaning:** "Hamahiga's sai."
- **Modern Interpretations:** Island/toponym-based eponym.
- **Conflicting Ideas & Origins:** Notationally stable.

The name "Hama Higa no Sai" (浜比嘉の釵) intricately intertwines geography, weaponry, and the rich cultural traditions of Okinawa's martial arts. The first part, "Hamahiga" (浜比嘉), refers to Hamahiga Island, a small yet spiritually significant isle in the Yokatsu archipelago off the eastern coast of Okinawa. Beyond its stunning beaches, the island holds deep importance in Ryukyuan cosmology, associated with sacred sites and creation myths that establish it as a cultural landmark. By naming the kata after this location, practitioners root their practice in a specific regional identity, which is a defining feature of Okinawan martial arts where place and technique are intrinsically connected.

The second component, "Sai" (釵), denotes the iconic iron truncheon, a weapon of Chinese origin likely inspired by "iron rulers," which Okinawa adapted into a versatile tool of kobudō. Used by law enforcement officials, such as the ufuchiku, to subdue opponents, the sai became emblematic of the Ryukyu Kingdom's ability to blend foreign influences with local needs. Its inclusion in the kata's name highlights its dual role as both a practical defensive tool and a cultural symbol.

The name carries historical significance through two figures associated with "Hama Higa." The first, Hama Higa Pechin (1663–1738), was a martial artist who demonstrated todi and saijutsu before Japan's 5th Tokugawa Shogun, Tsunayoshi, and even played Go with the famous master Honinbo Dosaku, showcasing his diverse talents. The second, Matsu Higa (1790–1870), is recognized for codifying kata for sai, tonfa, and bo in the 19th century. While oral traditions sometimes blur the lines between these individuals, their distinct timelines reflect separate contributions, with their legacies converging in the enduring name of the kata.

Hama Higa no Sai, preserved within lineages like Matsumura Seito's Kenshinkan branch under Fusei Kise and his son Isao Kise, represents more than just a name; it binds weapon practice to a place, honors Okinawa's martial heritage, and maintains a complex history where geography, identity, and artistry converge.

Hama Higa no Sai's Historical Roots

The exact origins of Hama Higa no Sai are shrouded in the complexities of Okinawan oral tradition. However, the story of this kata can be traced through two key figures whose legacies are intertwined.

The first figure is Hama Higa Pechin (1663–1738), a nobleman from Hamahiga Island known for his mastery of weaponry. Historical accounts describe him demonstrating todi and saijutsu before the Tokugawa shogun in Edo, showcasing the prestige of Ryukyuan martial skills. In addition to his martial talents, he gained recognition for winning a celebrated Go match against the legendary player Honinbo Dosaku, highlighting his scholarly acumen. Some traditions even suggest he studied under the Chinese envoy Wang Ji, known in Okinawa as Wanshu, who arrived in 1683. While the extent of this exchange is uncertain, it reflects the rich cross-cultural interactions of that period.

A century later, Matsu Higa (1790–1870), who is sometimes conflated with his predecessor, emerged as a pivotal figure in the codification of weapons kata. He is credited with formalizing techniques for the sai, tonfa, and bō, helping ensure their transmission during a time when Okinawan martial culture was being reshaped under Satsuma influence. It remains unclear whether Hama Higa no Sai was directly created by either man, named in their honor, or named after the island itself. What is evident is that both figures represent a blend of innovation and preservation that characterizes Okinawan martial tradition.

The development of the kata likely began in the late 17th to early 18th century, during the Ryukyu Kingdom's active tributary ties with China and Japan. Its refinement in the 19th century reflects the pressures of the Satsuma-controlled era, when the codification of weapon practices became increasingly important. This form effectively preserved practical sai techniques for the Pechin class, balancing defensive applications with the ceremonial value of public demonstrations.

Influenced by Chinese iron truncheon methods but distinctly Okinawan in character, Hama Higa no Sai exemplifies the adaptive spirit of Ryukyuan kobudō, melding external influences with local ingenuity to create a weapon tradition deeply connected to its place and people.

Applying Hama Higa no Sai's Combat Wisdom

Hama Higa no Sai embodies the balance of stability, adaptability, and precision that defines Okinawan weapon kata. Its stances, movements, and applications reveal not only practical combat strategies but also deeper principles of kobudō pedagogy.

At its core, the kata emphasizes rooted power through stances such as shiko-dachi (wide horse stance) and neko-ashi-dachi (cat stance), which provide both stability and mobility. Practitioners shift fluidly between grounded positions and higher, one-legged stances like tsuru-dachi (crane stance), demonstrating a tactical control of distance. These transitions highlight the dual demands of firmness and agility in weapon combat, allowing practitioners to absorb pressure and move closer or retreat as needed.

Technically, the sai is regarded not as an accessory but as an extension of the body. Strikes and parries reflect movements from empty-hand karate, reinforcing the integration of weapon and body mechanics. Key applications focus on neutralizing longer weapons, particularly the sword and bo. Targeting the hands, joints, and collarbones disrupts an opponent's grip or structure, creating decisive openings. A hallmark example is the "heaven and earth" block, where one sai guards high while the other protects low, effectively intercepting linear attacks. Success in such techniques relies more on refined wrist control, forearm alignment, and whole-body coordination than on brute strength.

Another layer of sophistication lies in the sai's versatility. Practitioners alternate between standard and reverse grips, using the yoku (prongs) to hook, trap, or strip weapons. This tactical variety underscores the adaptability that is highly valued in Okinawan kobudō. Equally important is the kata's reflection of the Ryukyuan ethic of measured response; the philosophy of force escalation. Students learn to calibrate their techniques, moving from controlled blocks to decisive disabling strikes, reflecting a humane martial approach that seeks resolution without unnecessary destruction.

Ultimately, the power of Hama Higa no Sai arises from efficient, integrated body mechanics, where hips, shoulders, and torsion work in harmony with stance and intention. More than just a collection of techniques, the kata conveys principles of timing, control, and adaptability that continue to embody the ingenuity of Okinawan martial practice.

Hama Higa no Sai's Evolving Traditions

Like many Okinawan kata, Hama Higa no Sai has evolved through various layers of transmission, adaptation, and interpretation. Its roots likely lie within the Pechin class, which preserved and practiced weapon traditions before the form was codified in the 19th century, most often attributed to Matsu Higa. From there, the kata was integrated into regional kobudō lineages, where it became closely tied to ideas of identity and heritage.

Despite a shared foundation, the kata today exhibits notable stylistic variations across different schools. One area of divergence is tempo: some traditions favor rapid, almost explosive execution with quick transitions and fast strikes, while others emphasize a more deliberate pace, grounded power, and precise technique. Body mechanics also vary. Certain versions highlight pronounced hip rotation to generate torque and fluidity, whereas others focus on compact power driven from the core and shoulders. The emphasis on stances can differ as well, featuring deep shiko-dachi for stability and strength or higher, more natural postures that favor agility and quick footwork.

Interpretations of bunkai reflect similar diversity. Some schools emphasize the sai's ability to trap, disarm, and control an opponent, while others concentrate more on striking or defensive counters against a sword or bo staff. Lineages also vary in how they structure continuity: some encourage seamless, flowing transitions, while others break movements into distinct segments, particularly for instructional clarity. For instance, Inoue Motokatsu's tradition emphasizes strong rooted stances, shoulder mechanics, and refined wrist control. In contrast, the Kenshinkan line, influenced by Matsumura Seito karate, favors crisp execution, speed, and a sharper integration of karate's body mechanics, leading to a pragmatic and forceful interpretation.

The reasons for such variation are numerous, including teacher interpretation, pedagogical emphasis, and even adaptations for demonstrations and competition. Yet beneath these differences, the kata's essence remains consistent; it trains the sai as both a weapon and an extension of the body, honing distance control, precision, and decisive application.

While the direct influence of Hama Higa no Sai on later kata is not fully documented, it almost certainly shaped subsequent sai forms and kobudō pedagogy in Okinawa. Its enduring adaptability across traditions highlights both the resilience and flexibility of the Okinawan martial arts heritage.

Hama Higa no Sai's Lasting Impact

Hama Higa no Sai serves both as a martial art form and a cultural landmark, connecting practitioners to the history and identity of Hamahiga Island and its distinguished Pechin. It emerged during the 17th and 18th centuries in the Ryukyu Kingdom, reflecting the martial ethos of that time: rooted stances, efficient mechanics, and the sai used as seamless extensions of the body. The movements emphasize precision over force, exploiting vulnerabilities through balance, timing, and leverage, rather than relying solely on brute strength.

As the kata spread among different traditions, each lineage introduced stylistic variations while maintaining its fundamental principles. This adaptability highlights the resilience of Okinawan martial arts, where preservation and innovation coexist harmoniously.

Today, Hama Higa no Sai persists not only as a technical exercise but also as a vessel of Ryukyuan memory. Practicing it becomes a dialogue with the past, recalling the warrior-scholars and codifiers who shaped it, the island roots that named it, and the cultural values it continues to embody. By carrying forward this kata, modern practitioners preserve more than just technique; they maintain a living expression of Okinawa's history, identity, and spirit.

TSUKEN SHITAHAKU NO SAI
Okinawa's Coastal Sai Tradition

Introduction to Tsuken Shitahaku no Sai

Few kata in Okinawan kobudō carry the weight and mystique of Tsuken Shitahaku no Sai. Traditionally reserved for advanced practitioners, this kata is expansive in scope, technically demanding, and deeply layered in meaning. Its very name, "the sai of Shitahaku from Tsuken," anchors it to the small island of Tsuken, a community long associated with skilled fighters and weapon specialists. Oral tradition holds that the form was composed by a 17th-century administrator of the Chinese embassy, whose position in Ryukyu placed him at the crossroads of politics, culture, and martial exchange. Whether myth or fact, this association underscores the kata's dual role as both a combat tool and a vessel of cultural memory.

As one of the five classical saijutsu kata, alongside Matsu Higa no Sai, Tawada no Sai, Chatan Yara no Sai, and Hamahiga no Sai, Tsuken Shitahaku no Sai occupies a central place in Okinawan weapons training. Within the Taira Shinken lineage, it has been preserved and transmitted as a cornerstone of traditional kobudō.

This chapter explores the kata's origins, technical intricacies, and layers of interpretation. It traces its transmission within Ryukyu Kobujutsu, highlights its role in shaping advanced sai practice, and critically distinguishes between documented history and the oral lore that surrounds it. In doing so, Tsuken Shitahaku no Sai emerges not merely as a demanding form, but as a cultural artifact, bridging island identity, Chinese influence, and Okinawan martial heritage.

Exploring the Essence of Tsuken Shitahaku no Sai

- **Traditional Notation:** 津堅志多伯の釵 (common modern writing); sometimes 下泊 used for the place "Shitahaku."
- **Script Breakdown:**
  - 津堅 "Tsuken";
  - 志多伯/下泊 "Shitahaku" (locality);
  - の posessive;
  - 釵 "sai."
- **Core Meaning:** "Sai of Tsuken–Shitahaku."
- **Modern Interpretations:** Taira Shinken lines preserve the toponym.
- **Conflicting Ideas & Origins:** Variant kanji for "Shitahaku" reflect different local spellings.

The name "Tsuken Shitahaku no Sai" holds significant historical and cultural meaning. The term "Tsuken" refers to Tsuken Island, a small but significant isle located southeast of Okinawa's main island, which has long been associated with fishing, maritime trade, and unique martial traditions. The second part, "Shitahaku," designates a real historical figure, an administrator or magistrate linked to the Chinese embassy in Naha around 1682. This identity firmly places the origins of the kata within the context of the Ryukyu Kingdom's diplomacy and governance, highlighting the connection between martial practices and civil service, along with cultural exchanges with China. The final term, "Sai," identifies the weapon central to the kata, an iron truncheon that was historically used for policing, defense, and as a symbol of authority.

Together, these elements create more than just a name; they encapsulate geography, individual legacy, and weaponry into a single expression. The use of kanji rather than phonetic transcription emphasizes the kata's Okinawan-Japanese authenticity while also reflecting the diverse cultural interactions present in the Ryukyu court. By connecting person and place, linking the heritage of Tsuken Island with Shitahaku's administrative role, the title situates the kata within a martial culture that is distinctly local yet heavily influenced by broader regional dynamics. In this way, "Tsuken Shitahaku no Sai" serves not just as a kata but as a historical statement, a living reminder of the Ryukyu Kingdom's unique fusion of geography, governance, and martial tradition.

Tsuken Shitahaku no Sai's Historical Roots

The kata has its origins in the late 17th century, during a time when the Ryukyu Kingdom was influenced by both Chinese and Japanese cultures. Its creation is attributed to Sai Taku, who is better known to modern practitioners by his Japanese name and title, Shitahaku Oyakata. He was born in Kumemura on January 4, 1645, and belonged to a distinguished lineage linked to Cai Xiang, a renowned scholar from the Song Dynasty. Shitahaku gained recognition as a high-ranking administrator.

Throughout his career, Shitahaku served as the Magistrate of Tsuken Island, a role that likely shaped his perspective on martial arts. In 1682, he was appointed the general administrator for the Chinese minister in Kume Village, where he oversaw diplomacy and trade with Qing China. These positions provided him with unique insights into both Ryukyuan and Chinese martial traditions. It was in this context that he is believed to have developed the techniques that became known as Tsuken Shitahaku no Sai.

Like other classical sai kata, its foundations stem from the adaptation of Chinese weapon techniques to Okinawan martial practice. However, Shitahaku's contribution extended beyond mere imitation; it involved codification. Utilizing the diverse influences available to him, he compiled a comprehensive repertoire of sai techniques that balanced practicality with a structured pedagogical approach. His work served multiple purposes; self-defense, skill display, and the training of future officials, aiming to preserve and transmit a disciplined martial system.

As part of a broader trend of kata development during the tributary age of the Ryukyu Kingdom, Tsuken Shitahaku no Sai is not only a product of its time but also a testament to the synthesis of cultures and the lasting legacy of kobudō as both a practice and a tradition.

Applying Tsuken Shitahaku no Sai's Combat Wisdom

At its core, Tsuken Shitahaku no Sai is a study of balance, stamina, and precision. The kata requires seamless transitions through a range of classical stances, including cat, front, horse, and crane. Each stance demands dynamic control while maintaining a stable foundation. These shifting positions reflect the kata's broader theme: the adaptability under pressure and the ability to flow between a rooted defense and an explosive offense.

The techniques in this kata form a diverse and challenging arsenal. Characteristic movements include vertical flips of the sai, crossing blocks that also serve as counterstrikes, sharp attacks to the temple and collarbone, and paired thrusts aimed at both high and low targets simultaneously. These applications not only showcase the weapon's versatility but also highlight its role in exploiting an opponent's blind spots. The mechanics behind these actions rely on generating power from the core, with fluid retraction and extension that provide both speed and control. Equally important is the precise wrist articulation that enables a practitioner to trap, deflect, or strike with surgical accuracy.

Beneath this technical repertoire lies a demanding internal dimension. The kata's length and complexity require stamina, focus, and breath control, embodying the principle of continuous, linked motion that characterizes much of traditional kobujutsu training. Through this combination of physical mechanics and internal discipline, Tsuken Shitahaku no Sai serves as both a test of endurance and a demonstration of the sai's potential as a weapon of adaptability and dominance.

Tsuken Shitahaku no Sai's Evolving Traditions

The transmission of Tsuken Shitahaku no Sai exemplifies both the continuity and adaptability inherent in Okinawan kobudō. This kata has been preserved through the efforts of masters such as Taira Shinken, who systematized weapon kata to ensure their survival into the modern era. Today, it appears in the curricula of various traditions, including Matayoshi Kobudō, Tokushin-ryu, and Ufuchiku Kobudō. The latter was established by Kanagusuku Sanda and further developed by practitioners like Shosei Kina, demonstrating that this kata has not only been inherited but also actively cultivated within broader weapons systems.

While the core structure of the kata remains recognizable across different lineages, small but significant stylistic differences have emerged. For example, in the Taira/Akamine lineage, practitioners tend to hold the tins of the sai horizontally when blocking, creating a whipping motion powered by the hips. In contrast, the Toon-ryu interpretation favors a vertical orientation, where the elbow is bent to allow for an explosive extension of the weapon. Such variations do not change the essence of the kata but rather express different pedagogical priorities, such as an emphasis on fluidity, power generation, or tactical clarity.

These refinements also illustrate how kata have evolved to meet the needs of practitioners and the demands of their eras. Some changes reflect the physical attributes of instructors or the requirements of modern teaching and demonstration, while others highlight interpretive choices made to preserve the kata's relevance without undermining its intent. Consistently across all traditions, the underlying character of the kata remains evident: it is a study in efficient trapping, decisive strikes, and the integration of hip-driven power.

As one of the classical sai kata, Tsuken Shitahaku no Sai continues to influence kobudō teaching beyond its own boundaries. Its principles can be seen in hybridized forms created by modern schools, and its techniques inform the broader language of Okinawan weaponry. Thus, the kata serves as both a vessel of continuity and a quiet innovator, linking the past to the present in the ongoing evolution of Okinawan martial practice.

Tsuken Shitahaku no Sai's Lasting Impact

Tsuken Shitahaku no Sai is not just a challenging sequence of techniques; it represents a living piece of Ryukyu's martial and cultural heritage. Originating from a 17th-century Tsuken Island official and shaped during a time of significant exchange, this kata preserves intricate mechanics, layered rhythms, and tactical nuances that reward only the most dedicated practitioners. Although variations have emerged across different lineages, its core structure has remained intact, ensuring that the kata is both historically significant and martially relevant today.

Practicing Tsuken Shitahaku no Sai allows one to follow in the footsteps of Okinawan officials and warriors, perpetuating a tradition that links diplomacy, administration, and kobudō. In this way, the kata continues to serve as a crucial connection between the living practice of Okinawan martial arts and its historical legacy.

TAWADA NO SAI
Okinawa's Tawada Line of Iron Trident

Introduction to Tawada no Sai

Ask a room full of seasoned kobudō practitioners which sai kata most rigorously requires coordination of weight, grip, and footwork, many will likely point to Tawada no Sai. This form is devoid of excess and ceremony, demanding precision without being showy, functioning more like a courtroom than a theatrical performance. It serves as a proving ground for serious, honest practice.

Though its emergence in the late 19th century marks it as one of the newest of the group, Tawada no Sai is widely regarded as one of the classical Okinawan saijutsu forms; including Chatan Yara no Sai, Tsuken Shitahaku no Sai, Hamahiga no Sai, and Matsu Higa no Sai. characterized by fluid transitions, powerful thrusts, and defensive maneuvers with the sai, often incorporating a third sai for advanced variations.

This chapter will explore what can be confidently stated about the kata, including its attribution to Tawada Shinzaku, its technical contributions to practical saijutsu, and its preservation and variations within Taira-line traditions and beyond. Where possible, we will differentiate between verifiable history and oral tradition, positioning Tawada no Sai as both a demanding training tool and an important link in the broader evolution of Okinawan kobudō.

Exploring the Essence of Tawada no Sai

- **Traditional Notation:** 多和田の釵.
- **Script Breakdown:**
  - 多和田 (Tawada, surname/toponym);
  - の posessive;
  - 釵 "sai."
- **Core Meaning:** "Tawada's sai."
- **Modern Interpretations:** Eponymic; appears in Taira/Matayoshi lines.
- **Conflicting Ideas & Origins:** Minor.

The name "Tawada no Sai" (多和田の釵) can be broken down into three components: "Tawada" (多和田), which is a family name of Okinawan origin; "no" (の), a genitive marker that means "of"; and "sai" (釵), a distinctive, truncheon-like weapon with side prongs that was historically used in law enforcement and civilian defense across the Ryukyus. Therefore, the title can be interpreted as "Tawada's sai" or "the sai of the Tawada lineage." The use of kanji instead of katakana emphasizes a strong domestic association, rooting the name within Okinawan cultural and linguistic traditions rather than implying foreign origins.

Most modern sources interpret "Tawada" as referring specifically to an individual, Tawada Shinzaku (sometimes spelled Shinjaku or Shinboku), who was an Okinawan martial artist and a student of Matsumura Sokon, active during the late nineteenth century. There is no direct documentary evidence from the Ryukyu Kingdom or early Meiji period that names the kata, so this connection relies on oral traditions that were later compiled and systematized in the twentieth century by Taira Shinken and his successors. It is important to note that the absence of primary records is neither unusual nor suspicious, as many classical kobudō kata have survived solely through teacher-to-student transmission rather than written catalogs.

In Okinawan martial culture, attaching a family name to a kata is significant. It indicates either authorship or a distinctive refinement of the practice, encoding both the provenance and accountability of the form. In a society where techniques were shared among village guards, court officials, and police constables, a name like "Tawada no Sai" not only identifies the individual who shaped the form but also reflects how it was remembered: as the unique way the Tawada family practiced the sai, thereby making it worthy of preservation under their name.

Tawada no Sai's Historical Roots

The origins of Tawada no Sai are traditionally linked to Tawada Pechin Shinkatsu, an aristocratic scholar-official in the Ryukyu Kingdom. The title "Pechin" indicated his position within the Ryukyuan caste system, a stratum responsible for administration, diplomacy, and security; roles that were somewhat similar to the samurai class in mainland Japan. Tawada was born during the kingdom's final decades of independence and lived through its annexation by Japan in 1879, a period marked by significant political and cultural change. In this evolving context, martial traditions once connected to royal service began to transition into private instruction and eventually into public training halls.

As is the case with many figures in nineteenth-century Okinawan martial culture, the details of Tawada's life remain scarce. However, lineage charts consistently credit him with shaping or transmitting the kata that bears his name. His training was influenced by prominent teachers: Matsumura Sokon, the renowned bodyguard to the last three Ryukyu kings and founder of Shuri-te, and the lesser-known Aburaya, who was recognized for his proficiency with the sai. From Matsumura, Tawada inherited a broad strategic understanding of Shuri-te and its weapon applications; from Aburaya, he likely absorbed specialized techniques related to saijutsu. This combination of influences is thought to have shaped the compact, guard-oriented tactics preserved in Tawada no Sai.

Given that Tawada lived in the late nineteenth century, it is important not to project the kata's origins further back in history without evidence. Although the sai had long been used by Ryukyuan constables (ufuchiku) for control, interception, and non-lethal strikes, there are no records indicating that this specific form existed prior to Tawada's time. Instead, Tawada no Sai should be understood as a structured distillation of these policing and self-defense methods, organized into a kata for both practice and transmission.

Applying Tawada no Sai's Combat Wisdom

Tawada no Sai presents a compact yet demanding study in saijutsu, combining practical stances, fluid grip transitions, and a tactical framework of deflecting, seizing, and countering. Its design reflects both Okinawa's policing traditions and the broader kobudō synthesis that emerged in the late nineteenth and early twentieth centuries.

Movement throughout the kata alternates between grounded stances, such as shiko-dachi, and more natural walking steps. This allows for quick advances or withdrawals against longer weapons, like the bo. A low, stable center and engaged hips provide the structure needed to absorb impact, redirect force, and drive the sai's weight through abrupt grip changes and forearm-based defenses. Proper breath timing and hip rotation reinforce power delivery, enabling short, explosive bursts of energy rather than prolonged exertion.

Technically, the kata emphasizes three fundamental grips: honte-mochi (natural), gyakute-mochi (reverse), and tokushu-mochi (specialized). Smooth transitions between these grips are a hallmark of proficient execution, allowing practitioners to adapt seamlessly between defense, entrapment, and striking. The tines of the sai play a central role, designed not to clash with weapons but to intercept, deflect, and trap. Once control is established, follow-up actions can include forearm crushes, wrist manipulations, or immediate counterstrikes.

Targeting follows the practical priorities of Okinawan law enforcement traditions: hands, wrists, elbows, and clavicles; these are joints and bony structures that can efficiently disable an opponent's weapon arm with minimal force. While there is some lore that credits the sai with the ability to "break swords," this should be viewed critically. Disrupting a cut or damaging lighter blades is plausible, but shattering a quality katana is far less realistic.

Strategically, the kata's sequences embody a measured rhythm of escalation: intercept the attack, seize control of the line, and respond with a decisive counter, whether it be a thrust, butt-end punch, or raking strike. In this respect, Tawada no Sai balances technical sophistication with a constabulary ethic: exercising restraint until necessary, followed by controlled and effective resolution. It is this fusion of mechanics, strategy, and cultural context that makes the form a cornerstone of advanced sai practice.

Tawada no Sai's Evolving Traditions

The journey of Tawada no Sai from a regional tradition to a staple of modern kobudō illustrates both careful preservation and creative adaptation. Tawada's students brought his teachings into the formative era of twentieth-century weapons practice, where Yabiku Moden incorporated the kata into his curriculum. From there, it passed to Taira Shinken, whose efforts to collect, standardize, and systematize Okinawan weapon forms ensured that Tawada no Sai would not be forgotten. Through Taira and his successors, such as Eisuke Akamine and Motokatsu Inoue, the kata spread beyond Okinawa, appearing in international lineages ranging from Matayoshi to Ufuchiku Kobudō, thereby establishing its place in the wider martial arts canon.

As the kata traveled, it inevitably evolved. Some lineages emphasize quick, close-range entries with restrained hip action, while others highlight larger stance shifts and a pronounced hip snap. The frequency and style of mochikae (grip changes) further distinguish these "house styles," confirming that no single authoritative version exists. These differences reflect various practical influences: some instructors simplify movements for accessibility, while others integrate karate-derived mechanics. Public demonstrations often prioritize rhythm and clarity over tactical subtlety. In modern saijutsu, Tawada no Sai plays a strategic role alongside companion forms such as Tsuken Shitahaku no Sai and Chatan Yara no Sai. Together, these forms provide a progression that develops range management, timing control, and increasingly sophisticated grip transitions, shaping the practitioner's understanding of the sai as both a weapon and an art. In this way, Tawada no Sai serves not only as a historical link to its originator but also as a living form that continues to evolve across different traditions.

Tawada no Sai's Lasting Impact

Attributed to Tawada Shinzaku, from the late nineteenth century, Tawada no Sai has been preserved and disseminated through the kobudō systematization led by Taira Shinken. While there is limited direct historical documentation, the kata's transmission across multiple lineages has ensured its survival and continued relevance.

Technically, the form emphasizes precise grip transitions, range management, and targeted strikes to the joints and forearms; core principles of effective sai usage. Over time, subtle variations have emerged within the Taira lineage and related schools, reflecting different pedagogical priorities, the integration of karate mechanics, and adaptations to various teaching contexts.

Today, Tawada no Sai serves as both a practical curriculum and a historical artifact. It trains practitioners to internalize the sai as an extension of their body, bridging civil order, self-defense, and disciplined martial practice. If Tsuken Shitahaku no Sai is akin to an epic novel, then Tawada no Sai resembles a legal brief: precise, procedural, and devastating when executed skillfully. Its study fosters honest movement, feet that are properly placed, hips that generate power, and hands that make critical decisions, allowing the iron to express itself.

MATSU HIGA NO SAI
Okinawa's Nimble Iron Fork

Introduction to Matsu Higa no Sai

Imagine a sai kata that is part technical manual, part island legend; a form credited to a diminutive yet formidable Pechin whose forearms were said to be "like tree trunks," strong enough to crush coconuts with his hands. That kata is Matsu Higa no Sai. Traditionally attributed to Matsu Higa Pechin, a semi-legendary figure celebrated for shaping structured methods of training in the sai, tonfa, and bo, the form embodies both combative utility and systematic pedagogy. Preserved within Taira Shinken's Ryukyu Kobudō system, it endures as a core kata, prized for its balance of practicality and clarity.

This chapter examines Matsu Higa no Sai through three interwoven perspectives: the historical and biographical background of Matsu Higa himself, the technical essence and stylistic influence of the form, and the transmission and interpretation of the kata across generations. Along the way, we will carefully distinguish legend from verifiable record, while situating the form within the broader martial and socio-political fabric of Okinawa. In doing so, Matsu Higa no Sai emerges not only as a training exercise but as a cultural artifact; an enduring testament to the resilience, ingenuity, and identity of Okinawan martial traditions.

Exploring the Essence of Matsu Higa no Sai

- **Traditional Notation:** 松比嘉の釵, (Matsu Higa no Sai)
- **Script Breakdown:**
    - 松比嘉 romanized variously as "Matsu Higa," or" Matsuhiga"
    - の posessive;
    - 釵 "sai."
- **Core Meaning:** "Matsuhiga's Sai."
- **Modern Interpretations:** Most modern historians treat him as a real but semi-legendary instructor, preserved mainly through weapon kata attribution..
- **Conflicting Ideas & Origins:** Name/reading confusion ("Matsuhiga" vs. "Matsu Higa") persists in English-language materials.

The name Matsu Higa no Sai (松比嘉の釵) encompasses multiple layers of meaning that go beyond the kata itself. The surname Matsu Higa (松比嘉) is connected to Hama Higa Island, indicating both a regional identity and a familial lineage. The particle "no" (の) serves as a genitive marker, translating to "of," which links the name to the weapon central to the kata: the sai (釵), an iron truncheon historically associated with Okinawan martial arts. This title effectively unites person, place, and weapon into a cohesive expression of heritage.

However, the historical figure behind the name is less clear. Popular accounts suggest that Matsu Higa was an 18th–19th century martial artist (circa 1790–1870), while other traditions point to an earlier Pechin of Hama Higa (1663–1738) who is said to have demonstrated martial techniques before the Shogun in Edo. The possibility that these figures or their deeds were conflated in later retellings complicates efforts to attribute the kata to one individual definitively.

Regardless of which Matsu Higa is associated with the name, it embodies more than mere authorship. It signifies accountability, linking the form to a lineage and a specific place. The sai itself serves as both a practical weapon and a cultural emblem, making Matsu Higa no Sai not just a name but a profound statement of legacy; a kata that is deeply rooted in Okinawa's martial heritage and passed down through the intricate interplay of memory, identity, and tradition.

Matsu Higa no Sai's Historical Roots

Matsu Higa no Sai is traditionally attributed to Matsu Higa Pechin (c. 1790–1870), an aristocratic guard from Hamahiga Island, located off the east coast of Okinawa. As a member of the pechin class, he lived during the declining years of the Ryukyu Kingdom, serving both as a civil official and a martial practitioner. Oral accounts describe him as compact yet immensely strong, standing barely over five feet tall, but capable of crushing coconuts with his hands and remaining undefeated in encounters with pirates and raiders. Such stories reflect the archetype of the Okinawan bushi: disciplined, pragmatic, and defined by a duty to protect.

The historical context, however, is complex. An earlier figure named Hama Higa Pechin (1663–1738) is recorded as demonstrating saijutsu before the Tokugawa Shogun in Edo, and some of his feats may be conflated with those attributed to the later Matsu Higa. Although their shared island origins and similar names can lead to confusion, most scholars conservatively date Matsu Higa no Sai to the 19th century, aligning it with the later figure's lifetime and the era's increasing emphasis on codifying martial practices.

Why was codification necessary at this point? Since 1609, the Ryukyu Kingdom had been under Satsuma overlordship, which restricted the open carriage of weapons but still required constabulary and village guards to maintain order. In this context, systematizing techniques using implements such as the sai, tonfa, and bo preserved practical methods and facilitated structured teaching. Matsu Higa no Sai embodies this dual purpose: it serves as both practical instruction for immediate use and a framework for passing knowledge to future generations.

Influence from Chinese martial traditions is also evident. Sources suggest that Matsu Higa studied under visiting emissaries and envoys, blending quan fa principles with indigenous methods. While no direct Chinese sai kata can be traced, the tactical logic: short-range redirection, joint targeting, and integration of empty-hand mechanics, demonstrates the hybrid character typical of Okinawan martial development.

Thus, the historical roots of Matsu Higa no Sai lie at the intersection of necessity and adaptation: a kata born from local duty, shaped by external influences, and preserved as a testament to the resilience of Ryukyuan martial culture during a time of significant political and social transition.

Applying Matsu Higa no Sai's Combat Wisdom

At the heart of Matsu Higa no Sai is an emphasis on stability, adaptability, and precision. The kata incorporates strong foundational stances that allow practitioners to root their weight while remaining capable of quick directional shifts. This balance between grounded power and fluid mobility is essential for effectively handling the sai, a weapon that requires both strength and finesse.

The technical execution within the kata highlights the sai's versatility through a variety of grips, expanding its defensive and offensive capabilities. Practitioners utilize blocks, traps, and swift counters, demonstrating the weapon's ability to control the rhythm of combat. A central aspect of sai methodology is using the weapon's tines to intercept and manipulate; this not only allows for catching an opponent's weapon but also enables practitioners to redirect or unbalance their movements. While folklore often describes the sai as capable of "snapping swords," historical and practical analysis reveal that its true strength lies in controlling limbs, destabilizing opponents, and striking vulnerable targets, such as the hands and wrists of adversaries wielding weapons.

The kata emphasizes a graduated response, beginning with redirection and restraint and escalating to decisive finishing strikes when necessary. This fluidity reflects the disciplined adaptability of kobudō, where restraint and control are valued equally with power and decisiveness. Underpinning this practice is the integration of rooted hip power, coordinated breathing, and a relaxed yet firm grip. This combination embodies the fusion of physical mechanics and mental composure that defines traditional Okinawan martial arts. Thus, Matsu Higa no Sai serves not only as a technical study of the weapon but also as a living expression of the broader kobudō philosophy: strength harmonized with precision and control balanced with resolve.

Matsu Higa no Sai's Evolving Traditions

Matsu Higa no Sai has primarily been preserved through the efforts of Taira Shinken, whose Ryukyu Kobudō system ensured that the kata was codified and passed down beyond oral tradition. From Taira's work in Okinawa, the form spread through his students, leading to international branches and securing its place as one of the core sai kata practiced today.

Like many classical weapon forms, Matsu Higa no Sai is not confined to a single "fixed" version. Instead, it exists in a range of interpretations that reflect the lineage and teaching objectives of different instructors. Some traditions emphasize crisp precision and strict adherence to form, while others focus on rooted power, fluidity, or even a touch of expressive flair. These variations often stem from differing goals, whether for educational clarity, practical combat application, or performance, as well as from how each teacher combines kobudō with karate mechanics or modern teaching methods.

Despite these differences, the kata remains central within the Matsu Higa weapons corpus. Practitioners often describe it as a structural backbone: a form whose mastery unlocks a deeper understanding of related kata and reveals the underlying principles that connect the series as a whole. In this sense, Matsu Higa no Sai is not merely a preserved relic of tradition, but rather a living thread that continues to unite the lineages of Okinawan kobudō practice.

Matsu Higa no Sai's Lasting Impact

Matsu Higa no Sai has been preserved mainly through the efforts of Taira Shinken, whose Ryukyu Kobudō system ensured that the kata was codified and passed down beyond oral tradition. Taira's work in Okinawa allowed the form to spread through his students into international branches, securing its position as one of the core sai kata practiced today.

Like many classical weapons forms, Matsu Higa no Sai is not limited to a single "fixed" version. Instead, it exists along a spectrum of interpretations that reflect the lineage and teaching methods of different instructors. Some traditions emphasize crisp precision and strict adherence to form, while others focus on rooted power, fluidity, or a bit of expressive flair. These variations often stem from differing goals, whether for educational clarity, practical combat application, or performance, as well as how each teacher integrates kobudō with karate techniques or modern teaching approaches.

Despite these differences, the kata remains central to the Matsu Higa weapons collection. Practitioners often describe it as a structural backbone: a form whose mastery unlocks deeper insights into related kata and reveals the underlying principles that connect the series as a whole. In this way, Matsu Higa no Sai is not just a preserved relic of tradition; it is a living thread that continues to bind together the lineages of Okinawan kobudō practice.

Section III – Tonfa-jutsu Kata

Okinawa's Tonfa: Turning Tools into Tactics

The sai is a short, trident-shaped iron weapon known for its unique defensive capabilities. While it is often associated with Japanese police tools, in Okinawa, it has been adapted for both civil defense and martial arts training. Its origins may trace back to Southeast Asian and Chinese weapons. Still, Okinawan tradition firmly establishes it within the Ryukyuan martial repertoire during the kingdom's maritime trade era.

The sai is particularly effective for trapping, parrying, and disarming opponents wielding weapons such as swords or staffs. It can also deliver thrusts and blunt strikes. In Okinawan culture, the sai symbolizes order and control; it is a weapon that neutralizes an opponent's advantage while embodying the disciplined, defensive spirit of martial arts. Its significance in kata demonstrates the Ryukyuan ability to combine practicality with cultural symbolism.

YARAGUWAA NO TONFA
Okinawa's Yara Family Tonfa Legacy

Introduction to Yaraguwaa no Tonfa

Few kata capture the imagination quite like Yaraguwaa no Tonfa. This form showcases the unique reverse grip of paired batons. Depending on whom you ask, this kata, which exists at the intersection of folklore, law enforcement practices, and praiseicle weaponry, is attributed either to a legendary Okinawan master or his talented son. Performed with a pair of tonfa (sometimes spelled tunfa or tuifa), which are short wooden batons with perpendicular side handles located about one-third of the way down the shaft, the form highlights ambidexterity, deflection-while-striking tactics, and compact circular power. These attributes made tonfa a practical choice for law enforcement and security roles in the Ryukyu Kingdom, and they remain central to the kata's identity today.

In modern Ryukyuan kobudō curricula, Yaraguwaa no Tonfa holds a significant position as one of the core tonfa forms, particularly within lineages that trace back to Taira Shinken. However, its history is shrouded in ambiguity. The name "Yaraguwaa" may serve as a diminutive nickname within the Yara family, adding to the ongoing debate about whether the kata should be credited to the well-known Chatan Yara or a lesser-known descendant. This chapter examines these historical questions while analyzing the form's technical characteristics, its reverse-grip mechanics, its simultaneous block-strike logic, and its transmission through documented teaching methods and oral traditions.

Exploring the Essence of Yaraguwaa no Tonfa

- **Traditional Notation:** 屋良小のトンファー / トゥンファー (Yara-gwā "Little Yara").
- **Script Breakdown:**
  - 屋良 "Yara";
  - 小 "small/young" (gwā diminutive);
  - の posessive;
  - トンファー tunfa / tonfa.
- **Core Meaning:** "(Little) Yara's tonfa."
- **Modern Interpretations:** Linked to Yara Guwa (son/disciple of Chatan Yara), or possibly the Yara family in general.
- **Conflicting Ideas & Origins:** Stable title; performed with Okinawan phonology in some schools.

The name Yaraguwaa (屋良小) combines "Yara" with the Uchinaaguchi diminutive suffix "-gwaa," which conveys meanings such as "little," "junior," or an affectionate nickname. Therefore, "Yaraguwaa no Tonfa" can be interpreted as "Little Yara's tonfa." The weapon is referred to in Japanese sources as "tonfa," which is a modern borrowing, or as "tuifa," which more accurately reflects the Okinawan pronunciation.

Modern literature from practitioners offers two main interpretations of the diminutive. One interpretation suggests that "Yaraguwaa" refers to Chatan Yara himself, possibly as a youthful or affectionate nickname. Another interpretation proposes that the kata commemorates Yara's son, to whom some contemporary retellings of Yara lore attribute the form. While this "son hypothesis" is frequently repeated in popular summaries, it lacks supporting evidence in historical Ryukyuan records, leaving its validity uncertain.

Regardless of which interpretation is correct, the name exemplifies a lasting tradition in Okinawa: kata are often named after families, teachers, or specific locations. The diminutive in this case suggests a personalized, house-style creation, illustrating the Yara family's distinctive approach to the tonfa within the broader kobudō repertoire.

Yaraguwaa no Tonfa's Historical Roots

Attributions connected to Chatan Yara, or to a descendant known as "Little Yara," fall into a gray area where folklore and identity intersect. The Yara figure plays a significant role in Okinawan weapon lore, and the name aligns with local naming conventions. However, no contemporary Ryukyuan records have definitively associated any tonfa kata with him. In other words, there is plausible heritage, but unproven authorship.

The name implies a direct connection to the historical Yara of Chatan, and the form incorporates techniques that recall an earlier time. However, the earliest confirmed record of Yaraguwaa no Tonfa is modern. It first emerged in print and organized teaching through the postwar systematization of Ryukyuan kobudō by Taira Shinken and the educational work of Inoue Motokatsu. Inoue's multi-volume work on Ryukyu Kobudō explicitly documents Yara Gwa no Tonfa, providing the first widely accessible account of the form. Meanwhile, Taira's efforts in the 1950s and 1960s to codify and promote kobudō laid the groundwork for its wider dissemination.

From that point forward, the kata became institutional rather than anecdotal; it features in the training lists of organizations and dojo lineages that trace back to Taira and Inoue, establishing a continuous and verifiable practice lineage rather than relying solely on oral tradition.

In summary, Yaraguwaa no Tonfa is best understood as a kata anchored in the mid-20th century, linked to Taira and Inoue, but also rooted in older traditions that connect it to history. This perspective allows us to appreciate the romance of the form while remaining honest about the historical record.

Applying the Yaraguwaa no Tonfa's Combat Wisdom

In Yaraguwaa no Tonfa, the weapon does not lead the motion; instead, the body drives, causing the tonfa to follow. The kata's power stems from the frame, with rooted pressure through the feet and the hips snapping and settling, allowing each strike or deflection to utilize the body's structure rather than relying solely on arm strength. The footwork emphasizes lateral stability and angular control, featuring wide, rooted stances like shiko-dachi in some lineages or forward-backward weight shifts from zenkutsu to kokutsu and back. Although stances may vary by school, their common goal remains the same: to achieve balance, redirection, and the generation of short, explosive power.

A defining feature of this form is the deliberate cycling through three tonfa grips: honte-mochi (natural grip), gyakute-mochi (reverse grip), and tokushu-mochi (shaft grip). Spending extended time in reverse grip develops close-range torque powered by the elbow and shoulder girdle. In contrast, rapid transitions between grips enhance dexterity and timing under pressure.

The kata emphasizes the tokushu-mochi grip as a signature flourish, using a flip to a shaft grip that transforms the side-handle into a functional hook. This grip facilitates snags, pulls, and rotational off-balancing, similar to kama tie-ups, and pairs well to convert catches directly into strikes. While the frequency of this maneuver may vary among lineages, its tactical logic reflects the kata's broader design.

In this kata, offensive and defensive actions are inseparable. The guard shapes are designed to strike; the edges, ridges, butt, and tip of the tonfa trace compact arcs that simultaneously deflect and counter. The governing principle is circular; tight redirections shed heavier lines of attack, such as a staff or sword cut, while feeding your own entry. Elbows stay close to conserve balance, turning the opponent's attack line into a bridge for your counterstrike. Breathwork and kime support this flow: inhale during loading, exhale sharply on impact, but never "freeze." In this context, kime represents the crisp punctuation of a moment, followed by an immediate transition into the next movement.

The bunkai themes across lineages share consistent motifs. When facing long weapons or extended strikes, practitioners often engage during the opponent's recovery, jamming the forearm or weapon shaft, torquing with the handle, and delivering immediate butt-end or shaft strikes to vulnerable targets. Simultaneity is crucial; blocking while hitting eliminates any gap between defense and offense. Hooks and traps from tokushu-mochi create takedown opportunities or safe exits. These body mechanics translate seamlessly to empty-hand techniques like uraken (back fist), hiji-waza (elbows), and forearm shields, highlighting the kata's potential historical role as a bridge between armed and unarmed close-range techniques.

Yaraguwaa no Tonfa's Evolving Traditions

The earliest reliable documentation of the kata known as Yaraguwaa no Tonfa does not stem from the era of the Ryukyu Kingdom but rather from a postwar initiative aimed at preserving and systematizing Okinawan weapon arts. In the early 1970s, Inoue Motokatsu's multi-volume work, "Ryukyu Kobudō," included Yaraguwaa no Tonfa among the standard tonfa kata. This inclusion reflected his teacher Taira Shinken's mission to document and safeguard forms that were at risk of disappearing. Since then, this kata has remained a core component of the Taira-Inoue curriculum, particularly within modern organizations such as Shimbukan and Bunbukan, which trace their lineage directly to this editorial effort.

The Taira-derived version of the kata embodies a postwar ethos of preservation and education. It emphasizes short, crisp movements that utilize decisive hip-driven power and practical techniques, in line with Taira's broader synthesis of karate and kobudō. The paired tonfa movements highlight continuity and flow. However, in a punctuated manner, dynamic transitions occur with clear beats, featuring reverse and special-grip sequences along with principles of close-range jamming and striking. Some branches of this lineage even offer a teaching variation in which a section can be performed using kama instead of tonfa, creatively acknowledging the shared mechanics between Okinawan weapons.

Additionally, the kata exists within the Kyan Chotoku tradition, but with a slight but distinctly different interpretation. Kyan, renowned for his natural and graceful approach to karate and kobudō, transmitted a version that emphasizes uninterrupted circular flow, natural posture, and continuous timing rather than segmented power accents. While the Taira/Inoue interpretation reflects postwar editorial standardization and karate hip dynamics, Kyan's schools prioritize fluid grace and the rhythmic qualities of kobudō.

Furthermore, some schools within the Kenshinkan lineage of Matsumura Seito practice this kata with a focus on combat clarity, highlighting grappling or tuite applications when applying techniques using the special grip. Despite these variations, all interpretations share essential structural elements: the use of paired weapons, both reverse and special-grip sequences, and the kata's hallmark close-quarters applications.

These differences should not be viewed as evidence of corruption from an imagined "original" form but rather as signs of a living tradition. Like many Okinawan weapon forms, Yaraguwaa no Tonfa has evolved to its current state through teacher-to-student transmission, editorial synthesis, and adaptation to changing instructional contexts. Taira's body of work itself included contributions and refinements from his students. At the same time, Kyan's followers maintained his personal style in their kobudō practice, as did practitioners from the Kise lineage. Today's various performances should be understood as parallel, documented adaptations of a kata that was institutionalized in the 20th century and continues to evolve. This dynamic quality, rooted in the preservation of tradition but open to adaptation, is what keeps Okinawan kobudō vibrant.

The Lasting Impact of Yaraguwaa no Tonfa

Linguistically and culturally, the name "Yaraguwaa" signals a connection to family-centered authorship. It combines the name "Yara" with an Okinawan diminutive suffix (-gwa/-gwaa), reflecting a local practice of using proper names to convey meanings, character traits, or themes that go beyond their literal definitions. This results in interpretations like "Little Yara" or a familial style specific to the Yara lineage. This label offers a meaningful insight into the social origins of the kata, even though it does not, by itself, confirm an 18th-century provenance.

Technically, the kata provides a compact toolkit for close-range control. It involves techniques such as extended reverse-grip cycling, rapid transitions between grips (including the shaft-grip or tokushu-mochi), and a block-strike unity that allows for immediate counters following deflections. These mechanics are well-suited for short-weapon control and can be effectively applied in empty-hand situations. This explains why the form serves as both a weapons kata and a drill for close-quarters control.

In summary, Yaraguwaa no Tonfa is a concise, tested system of short-weapon control that connects Ryukyuan naming practices, mid-20th-century codification, and living dojo variations. Whether the name signifies a youthful Yara, a son's creation, or an affectionate family style, the practical message of the kata remains consistent and clear: maintain a close range, disrupt the opponent's line, and finish with efficiency.

HAMAHIGA NO TONFA
Okinawa's Island Tonfa Legacy

Introduction to Hamahiga no Tonfa

The name "Hamahiga no Tonfa" evokes the gentle sound of waves lapping against the sacred shores of Hamahiga Island, a treasure in the Ryukyu archipelago, where ancient beliefs linger in the salty air. This name not only refers to a kata associated with the tonfa but also highlights the significance of Hamahiga Island, connecting Okinawa's martial arts heritage to its spiritual landscape. It combines practical techniques with the lasting legacy of both place and tradition. Long regarded as a sacred island in local lore, Hamahiga is deeply intertwined with spirituality and ancestral heritage, making the name of the kata more than just a geographical reference.

Within the realm of Okinawan kobudō, Hamahiga no Tonfa holds a unique position. While it is primarily recognized as the only tonfa kata in Isshin-ryu karate-kobudō, it has also been preserved in other styles, including Kenshinkan Matsumura Seito Shorin-ryu. In the Isshin-ryu system, it serves as the sole representative of tonfa practice, offering distinct value to practitioners who seek a connection between traditional weapon training and the broader Isshin-ryu curriculum.

This chapter will explore the kata's cultural and linguistic foundations, its role in Isshin-ryu through the efforts of its founder, Shimabuku Tatsuo, its possible older antecedents, its technical and combative logic, and its evolution through transmission. By doing so, it will situate Hamahiga no Tonfa within the larger context of Okinawan weapon traditions while emphasizing its ongoing relevance for practitioners today. This chapter will highlight why Hamahiga no Tonfa continues to resonate with martial artists who study both the mechanics of the weapon and the cultural spirit that underlies it.

Exploring the Essence of Hamahiga no Tonfa

- **Traditional Notation:** 浜比嘉のトンファー/トゥイファー.
- **Script Breakdown:**
    - 浜比嘉 Island name
    - の posessive;
    - トンファー tunfa / tonfa.
- **Core Meaning:** "Hamahiga's tonfa."
- **Modern Interpretations:** Standard Matayoshi/Ryūkyū kobudō repertoire.
- **Conflicting Ideas & Origins:** None substantial.

The name "Hamahiga no Tonfa" (浜比嘉のトゥイファー / トンファー) is both linguistically clear and culturally significant. The term "Hamahiga" (浜比嘉) combines "hama" (浜), which means "beach" or "coast," with "Higa" (比嘉), a Ryukyuan surname and village name. Together, this compound refers to Hamahiga Island (Hamahiga-jima), a small yet symbolically rich island near Okinawa's Katsuren Peninsula. In Ryukyuan belief, Hamahiga is revered as a sacred place associated with creation myths and the worship of ancestors. This connection lends the kata's title cultural depth beyond its martial practice.

The second element, "tonfa" (トンファー or トゥイファー in katakana), refers to the side-handled wooden baton that has been codified as a kobudō weapon. Its phonetic rendering in katakana suggests a non-standard or regional origin, possibly stemming from Okinawan dialects or influences from the Chinese language. This reflects the cultural crosscurrents that have shaped Okinawan martial vocabulary.

Unlike some kata names that may invite debate over personal, symbolic, or abstract associations, "Hamahiga no Tonfa" is straightforward: it refers to a tonfa kata linked specifically to Hamahiga. However, the island's status as a site of spiritual significance adds a layer of meaning that elevates the name beyond mere geography. By associating the form with a place rich in Ryukyuan identity, the kata's title serves as both a martial curriculum element and a cultural marker, emblematic of the blending of combative practices and sacred traditions in Okinawa.

While the name firmly situates the kata within Okinawa's cultural and spiritual landscape, its historical origins as a codified form are more elusive.

Hamahiga no Tonfa's Historical Roots

The historical background of Hamahiga no Tonfa is a tapestry woven from documented figures, oral traditions, and modern preservation efforts. A key figure in this transmission is Taira Shinken, who dedicated himself to collecting and codifying Ryukyuan kobudō during the 20th century, ensuring the survival of many classical forms.

The origins of the tonfa are less specific but culturally significant. Two notable figures from Hamahiga Island with the Higa name often arise in discussions about the beginnings of modern kobudō. The first, Higa Pechin (1663–1738), is featured in Ryukyuan and Japanese records as a Go master and martial artist, demonstrating todi (empty hand) techniques and sai before Shogun Tokugawa Tsunayoshi in Edo. Although his documented expertise does not include the tonfa, his status as a Hamahiga-born pechin connects the island to a martial reputation. The second figure, Matsu Higa (1790–1870), another pechin, is credited in 20th-century sources, including Taira Shinken's writings, with codifying kata for the bo, sai, and tonfa.

The frequent confusion between these two Higa figures, who were separated by more than a century, likely stems from oral traditions that merged names and places into a single legendary source. Scholars like Andreas Quast and Patrick McCarthy observe that this blending reflects a broader trend in Okinawan martial historiography, where the lines between documented history and local memory often blur. Therefore, legends surrounding the kata's origins in Hamahiga may contain elements of truth, even if exact authorship remains elusive.

From a technical perspective, the kata's structure emphasizes fluid rotations, defensive sweeps, and strikes, aligning with the 19th-century movement to codify kobudō into teachable forms. References in works such as the Bugei Ryūha Daijiten (1978) confirm its acknowledgment within the Matayoshi and Taira lineages. However, whether Taira preserved an older form or reconstructed elements from regional practices remains uncertain. By the mid-20th century, the kata had been secured within Isshin-ryu through Shimabuku's adoption, ensuring its continuity into the modern era.

In summary, the roots of Hamahiga no Tonfa reveal a complex history that intertwines oral traditions connecting it to Hamahiga's pechin families, potential 19th-century codification, and 20th-century preservation. This interplay of legend, adaptation, and documentation exemplifies how many kobudō kata navigate the boundary between cultural heritage and the systematic organization of martial arts.

Applying Hamahiga no Tonfa's Combat Wisdom

At its core, Hamahiga no Tonfa represents a fusion of strong fundamental stances, precise body mechanics, and the unique versatility of paired tonfa. The form emphasizes stability and rootedness, with the Han-zenkutsu dachi (half-front stance) and Zenkutsu dachi providing balance for linear strikes and thrusts, while the Kiba dachi (horse stance) anchors powerful frontal techniques. These stances not only serve as postural frameworks but also as launch points for explosive transitions, sweeps, and counters. Breath control is interwoven throughout the kata, reinforcing both mental focus and the generation of whole-body power, a hallmark of Okinawan practice.

The kata enhances the practitioner's ability to integrate defense and offense in a seamless, flowing manner. Defensively, the tonfa extends and reinforces natural arm blocks. Techniques such as the vertical forearm block and rising block use the weapon as a shield against head- and collarbone-level strikes. In contrast, the tenchi-uke (heaven and earth block) provides layered coverage against simultaneous high and low attacks. These methods highlight the tonfa's dual role as both a guard and a lever, allowing for the redirection of force while setting up for counterstrikes.

Offensively, Hamahiga no Tonfa showcases the weapon's capacity for both blunt-force impact and continuous striking patterns. The figure-eight strike is a signature element that trains rhythm, coordination, and the ability to chain attacks across multiple planes. Horizontal sweeps at waist level, diagonal downward strikes, and thrusting actions mirror the mechanics of empty-hand techniques, while magnifying their effectiveness through the weight and leverage of the tonfa. The vertical "flip" action, where the weapon snaps upward into a ready position, exemplifies the kata's demand for dexterity and its emphasis on rapid transitions between guard and attack.

A notable principle woven throughout the kata is adaptability: a block is rarely an endpoint but rather the beginning of a sweep, strike, or lock. In some interpretations, a leg sweep is paired with a simultaneous counterstrike, illustrating how the kata conditions practitioners to blend striking, controlling, and unbalancing actions into a single, fluid sequence. The sharp clack of paired tonfa meeting during certain techniques serves not only as a tactical strike at neck or jaw height but also as an auditory cue of precision and timing.

Compared to other tonfa kata, such as Yaraguwaa no Tonfa, which emphasizes smaller circular motions and rapid transitions, Hamahiga no Tonfa tends to highlight stronger rooted stances and more pronounced figure-eight patterns, giving it a heavier, grounded character within the tonfa repertoire.

Together, these technical features reveal a kata designed not only to refine weapon mechanics but also to embody broader Okinawan kobudō principles of efficiency, adaptability, and integration. To fully understand how these methods have been preserved and adapted, we must next examine the history of the kata's transmission and the variations that have arisen across different lineages.

Hamahiga no Tonfa's Evolving Traditions

The transmission of Hamahiga no Tonfa illustrates both the oral traditions of Okinawa and the efforts to systematize these practices in the 20th century. For centuries, kobudō knowledge was passed down quietly within pechin families and local teachers, often without written records. It was Taira Shinken, known as the "Funakoshi of Kobudō," who took on the task of collecting, codifying, and preserving these forms. During his travels across Okinawa, Taira studied with masters such as Moden Yabiku and drew upon traditions associated with figures like Matsu Higa. He ultimately created a curriculum that organized tonfa, sai, bo, and other weapons into a coherent system. Within this framework, Hamahiga no Tonfa was preserved alongside Yaraguwaa no Tonfa. Taira's teachings shaped several important lines of transmission. Students like Motokatsu Inoue, who later established the Ryukyu Kobujutsu Hozon Shinkokai, played a crucial role in spreading the kata in Japan and abroad. Archival footage of Taira performing the form became a reference point for subsequent generations, standardizing its practice in international dojos worldwide.

The kata also entered the Isshin-ryu tradition through Tatsuo Shimabuku. Having founded Isshin-ryu in 1956, Shimabuku began studying kobudō under Taira in 1958, incorporating Hamahiga no Tonfa into his curriculum around 1960. It became Isshin-ryu's sole tonfa kata, which Shimabuku taught to first-generation students, including Arcenio Advincula, Angi Uezu, and Steve Armstrong. While Isshin-ryu's adaptation is somewhat more compact and closely integrated with karate's empty-hand principles, it preserved the kata as an essential link between weapon and unarmed practice.

Another line of transmission emerged in Kenshinkan Matsumura Seito Shorin-ryu. Fusei Kise established Kenshinkan in 1977 after extensive training with teachers such as Hohan Soken and Shigeru Nakamura. His son, who helped carry the system into the future, included Hamahiga no Tonfa in his kobudō curriculum, where it became a standard element of the All Okinawan Shorin-ryu Matsumura Seito Karate and Kobudō Federation (OSMKKF). Here, it is practiced with the linear precision and subtle hip mechanics characteristic of Matsumura Seito, often taught step-by-step with a strong focus on bunkai and close-quarters applications.

Across these lineages, stylistic differences reflect the priorities of each tradition. In the Taira line, the kata is expansive and fundamental, emphasizing large arcs, grip transitions, and building power through circular momentum, creating a style that feels "classical" in its preservationist approach. Isshin-ryu versions are shorter and more direct, structured with compact footwork, quick reversals, and practical counters that echo the system's empty-hand kata, such as Seisan. Kenshinkan practice, by contrast, is more combat-oriented, focusing on transitions, hip rotation, and integrating tuite principles within the flow of techniques.

Together, these variations reveal not divergence but adaptability: each branch retains the kata's core of fluid transitions, paired block-strike combinations, and characteristic figure-eight patterns, while shaping its practice to align with the pedagogical and combative philosophies of its respective systems. In this way, Hamahiga no Tonfa reflects the larger story of Okinawan kobudō: preservation through adaptation that ensures continuity while allowing expression across diverse lineages.

Hamahiga no Tonfa's Lasting Impact

Hamahiga no Tonfa combines cultural symbolism with martial function. Its name connects the kata to Hamahiga Island, a sacred site in Ryukyuan tradition, and its technical vocabulary demonstrates the versatility of the tonfa as both a shield and a striking weapon. Historically, this form reflects a rich heritage: oral traditions link it to the pechin families of Hamahiga, while its codification and preservation are primarily attributed to Taira Shinken, followed by its adoption by Tatsuo Shimabuku in Isshin-ryu, as well as the Kise family's Kenshinkan.

In terms of technique, the kata focuses on rooted stances, figure-eight patterns, and adaptability, training practitioners to seamlessly blend blocks, strikes, sweeps, and counters in a continuous flow. The variations of the kata across the Taira, Isshin-ryu, and Kenshinkan lineages illustrate a broader trend in Okinawa of preserving traditions through adaptation. Each branch retains the essence of the kata while refining it to align with its respective style.

Today, Hamahiga no Tonfa remains both a practical training form and a cultural repository. It preserves historical memory, imparts combative principles, and connects modern practitioners with the enduring spirit of Okinawan kobudō.

MATSU HIGA NO TONFA
Okinawa's Enduring Tonfa Heritage

Introduction to Matsu Higa no Tonfa

Many practitioners may not realize that Matsu Higa no Tonfa is more than just a dynamic weapons kata; it is named after a semi-legendary Okinawan warrior known for his remarkable strength and martial skills, which blur the lines between history and myth. This kata is part of the rich kobudō tradition, utilizing paired tonfa: side-handled wooden weapons that combine defense, control, and powerful striking techniques. Alongside Matsu Higa no Kon and Matsu Higa no Sai, it forms a trio of weapon forms attributed to Matsu Higa, who is celebrated in Okinawan lore as both a skilled fighter and a preserver of martial teachings.

In this context, Matsu Higa no Tonfa is valued not only for its effectiveness in combat but also for its role as a vessel of lineage, preserving techniques and principles across generations. This chapter will explore the kata's origins and its connection to its namesake, balancing historical evidence with oral tradition. It will examine its technical contributions, cultural significance, and transmission through various lineages. In doing so, the aim is to situate Matsu Higa no Tonfa within the broader framework of Okinawan martial heritage, where memory, myth, and practice converge.

Exploring the Essence of Matsu Higa no Tonfa

- **Traditional Notation:** 松比嘉のトンファー, (Matsu Higa no Tunfa)
- **Script Breakdown:**
  - 松比嘉 romanized variously as "Matsu Higa," or" Matsuhiga"
  - の posessive;
  - トンファー tunfa / tonfa.
- **Core Meaning:** "Matsuhiga's Tunfa."
- **Modern Interpretations:** Most modern historians treat him as a real but semi-legendary instructor, preserved mainly through weapon kata attribution..
- **Conflicting Ideas & Origins:** Name/reading confusion ("Matsuhiga" vs. "Matsu Higa") persists in English-language materials.

The name Matsu Higa no Tonfa (松比嘉のトンファー) is a simple yet culturally rich phrase that connects a legendary figure, a weapon, and a martial legacy. Breaking it down: Matsu Higa refers to a semi-legendary Okinawan martial artist associated with Hamahiga Island. He is remembered as a member of the Pechin class, which comprised the hereditary warrior-bureaucrat elite of the Ryukyu Kingdom. His name can be written as 松比嘉 or in dialectal form as マチュー・ヒジャー. The surname Higa is common in Okinawa, while Matsu (meaning "pine") symbolizes

195

endurance and resilience in Japanese culture. The particle "no" (の) indicates possession, translating the phrase to "the tonfa of Matsu Higa." The final element, Tonfa (トンファー), refers to the paired wooden side-handled weapon itself. Together, the title denotes this kata as the form of tonfa techniques attributed to Matsu Higa.

This choice to honor Matsu Higa in the kata's name recognizes his significance, whether historical or legendary, in systematizing weapons practice. He is traditionally credited with codifying forms for the bo, sai, and tonfa, while also transmitting techniques that were influenced by both indigenous Okinawan methods and Chinese martial systems. However, the precise details of his life are still debated. He is often conflated with Higa Peichin (1647–1721), an earlier figure from the same class, and the hereditary nature of the Pechin title has made generational boundaries less clear. This confusion has led to a mix-up between "Matsu Higa no Tonfa" and the similarly named Hamahiga no Tonfa, which is a separate kata of different origin.

Despite these uncertainties, the name itself firmly roots the kata within Okinawan martial heritage. It connects a specific weapon form to a cultural identity grounded in the Ryukyu Kingdom's warrior class, ensuring that both the legend of Matsu Higa and the practical combative lessons of the tonfa continue to be preserved in practice.

This story embedded in the name naturally leads us to explore the man and the moment behind it, raising questions of origin, context, and purpose that help define the historical roots of kata.

Matsu Higa no Tonfa's Historical Roots

The origins of Matsu Higa no Tonfa are closely tied to the semi-legendary figure of Matsu Higa, a martial artist from Hamahiga Island, often associated with the Pechin class, the hereditary warrior-bureaucrats of the Ryukyu Kingdom. Tradition credits him with codifying several weapon kata, including forms for the bo, sai, and tonfa. However, details of his biography are elusive; some accounts place him in the late 18th to 19th century (circa 1790–1870), while others conflate him with Higa Peichin (1647–1721), suggesting either a familial connection or confusion over generations. This uncertainty highlights the blend of oral tradition, myth, and fragmentary records that characterize much of Okinawa's martial heritage.

Although the kata's technical content likely dates back to an earlier period, the title Matsu Higa no Tonfa did not appear in written sources until the 20th century when kobudō was being systematically codified and popularized. Before this formalization, martial knowledge was primarily preserved orally and transmitted privately, often within families or between teachers and select students. The codification into kata was a practical response to the fragility of this transmission; it distilled combative principles into repeatable sequences that could be reliably passed down through generations. For Matsu Higa, the systematization of weapon forms helped ensure the survival of knowledge that might have otherwise been lost or diluted through informal transmission.

The motivations for codifying a kata such as Matsu Higa no Tonfa must be understood within the broader martial and social context of Okinawa. In a world where mistakes in combat could be fatal, techniques were prized for their efficiency and economy of motion. Legend states that Matsu Higa's methods were "fundamental and efficient, with no wasted movements," which would have made them practical for self-defense and memorable for instruction. By structuring these lessons into kata, he created a tool for training consistency and the preservation of lineage, ensuring that kobudō knowledge could endure despite the restrictions imposed by the Satsuma occupation and later Japanese rule.

Influences on the form likely extended beyond Okinawa itself. As a maritime hub, the Ryukyu Kingdom absorbed techniques and ideas from Chinese martial arts (quan fa), transmitted through envoys and resident experts such as Zhang Xue Li and Wang Ji. Elements of these Chinese systems were blended with indigenous Okinawan practices, resulting in hybrid forms that reflected both foreign inspiration and local adaptation. The tonfa is thought to have Southeast Asian or Chinese roots, although its connection to millstone handles provided a convenient Okinawan analogy. Within this cultural crossroads, Matsu Higa's synthesis of techniques into kata exemplifies how Ryukyuan martial traditions preserved, transformed, and transmitted knowledge across time and lineage.

While the historical record offers a glimpse into the legacy of Matsu Higa, it is in the kata's techniques and principles that his teachings come to life, revealing how theory, efficiency, and survival were distilled into movement.

Applying Matsu Higa no Tonfa's Combat Wisdom

At its core, Matsu Higa no Tonfa is a study in efficiency, combining both the defensive utility and offensive power of the tonfa into movements that are economical and decisive. The kata illustrates the weapon's adaptability, which can seamlessly transition from a shield to a striking implement. Additionally, it emphasizes the balance between rooted stability and fluid redirection. Each sequence demonstrates how Okinawan kobudō has distilled combat principles into repeatable forms that embody both physical technique and strategic philosophy.

The foundation of the kata lies in its stances, which provide the base from which all techniques flow. Zenkutsu dachi, or forward stance, dominates the form, delivering thrusts and blocks with committed momentum while maintaining balance through a solidly planted rear leg. In contrast, kiba dachi, the horse stance, emphasizes lateral stability, grounding the practitioner for strikes and low-level defenses that require immovable strength from the hips. Shiko dachi, with its wide, outward-turned footing and low center of gravity, supports dropping techniques like otoshi zuki, producing explosive downward power ideal for counters and finishing strikes. The use of sokutsu dachi, or side stance, highlights lateral mobility and the ability to shift weight quickly for alternating defenses such as tenchi uke. Meanwhile, heiko dachi, a neutral parallel stance, allows for rapid transitions into strikes or evasions without deep commitment. The appearance of tsuru ashi dachi, the one-legged crane stance, further refines the practitioner's balance, pairing stability with readiness for high-level defense or evasive kicking techniques. Together, these stances illustrate a rhythm of advance, anchoring, and redirection that lies at the heart of the kata's combative logic.

The technical repertoire of Matsu Higa no Tonfa reinforces the balance between defense and offense. Low sweeping blocks, or gedan uke, deflect attacks while clearing the way for immediate counterattacks, often executed with the extended shafts of the tonfa. The double forearm block, ude uke, performed with the weapons clapping audibly together, shields the upper line and chambers the arms for rapid follow-up strikes. The alternating high-and-low defense of tenchi uke, or "heaven and earth block," exemplifies the kata's emphasis on layered protection, training the practitioner to defend multiple levels simultaneously. From these defensive foundations flow a wide array of strikes: straight thrusts such as chudan zuki and gyaku zuki extend the practitioner's reach, while circular techniques like hachinoji furi generate continuous momentum for combinations that transition fluidly into vertical chops, horizontal swings, or overhead cleaves. The signature otoshi zuki, delivered from a deep shiko dachi, showcases the kata's intent to conclude engagements decisively, combining downward power with grounded stability to finish a subdued or fallen opponent.

Additional elements within the form expand its tactical vocabulary. Foot sweeps such as ashi bari disrupt balance before decisive follow-up strikes, while the subtle nami ashi, or "returning wave," introduces a rhythm of evasion and recovery early in the kata. Shifts in grip, from hon te-mochi (standard grip) to gyaku te-mochi (reverse grip) and back again, demonstrate the tonfa's versatility, allowing practitioners to adapt instantly between reinforced blocks, thrusts, and rotational swings. These transitions highlight the weapon's ability to serve as both shield and club, embodying the Okinawan principle that every movement should carry multiple combat possibilities.

Underlying all of these techniques are the deeper lessons of the kata. It demands rootedness, achieved through strong stances that channel the body's weight into each action, while equally insisting on adaptability, as seen in the fluid transitions and lateral movements that prevent rigidity. It emphasizes economy, ensuring that every block can double as a potential strike and every shift in position creates new tactical opportunities. This interplay of offense and defense, stability and motion, reflects the pragmatic nature of Okinawan martial culture, where survival depended not on elaborate techniques but on mastering the essentials delivered with precision.

In summary, Matsu Higa no Tonfa is not merely a catalog of movements but a comprehensive training method. Its structure teaches practitioners how to root themselves firmly while remaining fluid, how to defend and strike in the same motion, and how to wield the tonfa as an extension of both body and strategy. In doing so, the kata preserves not only the techniques of a legendary figure but also the enduring principles of Okinawan kobudō: efficiency, adaptability, and decisive action in the face of danger.

While the kata's techniques embody timeless principles of efficiency and adaptability, its survival owes much to the generations that have preserved and adapted it. The journey of this kata, preserved, adapted, and sometimes transformed, speaks to the resilience of Okinawan kobudō.

Matsu Higa no Tonfa's Evolving Traditions

Matsu Higa no Tonfa, like many weapon forms from Okinawa, was originally shared through oral transmission within the Pechin class, passed discreetly from teacher to student. The techniques were not documented until much later, when 20th-century preservationists, such as Taira Shinken, began collecting and codifying kobudō kata into structured curricula. By this time, Matsu Higa no Tonfa was recognized among classical Okinawan forms and was often listed alongside Hamahiga no Tonfa and Yaraguwa no Tonfa as part of a core group of tonfa kata. Today, this form is practiced in several traditions, including branches of Kanken Toyama's Shudokan lineage, Kenwa Mabuni's Shito-ryu, and advanced practitioners of Taira Shinken's Ryukyu Kobudō Shimbukan, ensuring its survival in both karate-focused and kobudō-centered schools.

As with many kata, the transmission of Matsu Higa no Tonfa has not been uniform, leading to stylistic variations over time. In systems dedicated specifically to kobudō, the form emphasizes the weapon's unique mechanics: fluid wrist and forearm rotations, reinforced blocking with the tonfa's shaft, and strikes that make deliberate use of the handle's extended tip. However, when practiced within karate-oriented lineages, the kata often reflects the dynamics of the originating system. For example, a Shorin-ryu approach might favor lighter, more natural stances with quick evasive movements, while a Shito-ryu rendition may incorporate the distinctive hip vibrations characteristic of that style.

In addition to these structural differences, subtler nuances also distinguish the kata across various schools. Variations in timing, tempo, and execution can be quite pronounced; one lineage might teach a slow, controlled rotation of the tonfa to emphasize precision, while another may perform the same movement as a sharp, snapping strike to highlight speed.

These variations do not diminish the kata's significance; rather, they showcase the vitality of Okinawan martial traditions, which have always balanced preservation with adaptation. In the case of Matsu Higa no Tonfa, this multiplicity of interpretations reflects both its deep historical roots and its ongoing relevance as a means for training, experimentation, and the expression of lineage identity.

The journey of Matsu Higa no Tonfa, from oral preservation to modern reinterpretation, illustrates both the fragility and resilience of Okinawan kobudō. To fully appreciate its significance, we must consider not only how it has been transmitted but also how it endures as a lasting symbol of martial wisdom and cultural identity.

Matsu Higa no Tonfa's Lasting Impact

The study of Matsu Higa no Tonfa reveals a kata that serves as both a vessel of history and a system of combative principles. Its name preserves the memory of a semi-legendary Pechin, grounding the form in both lineage and geography. These historical roots remind us of the delicate yet enduring nature of Okinawan oral traditions, while the techniques demonstrate a pragmatic blend of stability, fluidity, and efficiency that characterized Okinawan approaches to armed defense. The kata's evolution through different lineages highlights how adaptation and preservation have worked together to keep its teachings alive.

Today, the form endures as more than just a technical exercise. It serves as a training method that develops coordination, balance, and the practical application of the tonfa's unique mechanics. Additionally, it acts as a cultural artifact, linking practitioners to the martial traditions of the Ryukyu Kingdom and illustrating the process by which oral teachings became codified kata. In both karate-centric and kobudō-focused schools, the kata continues to bridge weapon practice with broader martial principles, embodying the values of efficiency, decisiveness, and adaptability. Looking ahead, the significance of Matsu Higa no Tonfa lies not only in its preservation but also in its role as a living tradition. Each generation that studies and interprets the kata contributes to its survival, ensuring that it remains relevant in practice while still connecting to its historical roots. In this way, the kata links modern practitioners to a legacy of resilience and ingenuity, serving as both a reminder of Okinawa's martial past and a guide for future study.

SECTION IV – NUNCHAKU-JUTSU KATA

Okinawa's Flails: Whirling Storm of Wood and Cord

Cnsisting of two short sticks connected by a cord or chain, the nunchaku are one of the most recognizable yet often misunderstood weapons from Okinawa. Many people see it as merely a theatrical or cinematic prop, but its traditional purpose is much more practical. The exact origins of the nunchaku are uncertain; some suggest a connection to Southern China, while others believe it was adapted from horse bridles or farm tools like flails.

In Okinawan kobudō, the nunchaku is used to cultivate skills in timing, distance, and rhythm. It teaches users how to control centrifugal force, redirect energy, and maintain a continuous flow of movement. These lessons emphasize adaptability and improvisation. The nunchaku's lasting role in kobudō embodies the Ryukyuan spirit of creativity and resilience, transforming a simple tool into a weapon that is both elegant and practical.

MATAYOSHI NO NUNCHAKU
Okinawa's Keeper of the Nunchaku Flame

Introduction to Matayoshi no Nunchaku

Few kobudō forms combine simplicity and depth quite like Matayoshi no Nunchaku. To those unfamiliar, the nunchaku may seem like merely two wooden sticks connected by a cord or chain, often dismissed as a mere flashy curiosity. However, within the Okinawan martial tradition, this seemingly humble tool serves as a means to explore crucial concepts such as timing, distance, rhythm, and mobility. Studying the nunchaku reveals not only its technical sophistication but also the creativity of a culture that transformed everyday tools into instruments of defense.

In the Matayoshi kobudō system, Matayoshi no Nunchaku is the primary formal kata for this flexible weapon, positioned as the fourth form in the official curriculum. Its structured sequences teach practitioners how to control the nunchaku's unpredictable arcs, integrate striking and blocking into a continuous flow, and adapt to both armed and unarmed opponents. As such, it acts as a bridge between basic familiarity with the weapon and the deeper combative and conceptual skills necessary for mastery, making it essential for a student's progression through the Matayoshi system.

This chapter will explore the historical roots and cultural context of Matayoshi no Nunchaku. It will examine the origins of the weapon and its adaptation from agricultural tools, the role of the Matayoshi family in preserving and transmitting its practice, the kata's technical structure and applications, and how its traditions have evolved across different lineages. Ultimately, it will assess the form's enduring legacy within modern kobudō, where it remains both a technical discipline and a cultural emblem of Okinawan resilience and creativity.

As with many Okinawan weapon forms, clarity begins with understanding the kata's name; the title Matayoshi no Nunchaku is itself a window into the cultural and familial legacy that frames its practice.

Exploring the Essence of Matayoshi no Nunchaku

- **Traditional Notation:** 又吉のヌンチャク (Matayoshi no Nunchaku).
- **Script Breakdown:**
    - 又吉 (Matayoshi, surname);
    - の posessive;
    - ヌンチャク nunchaku.
- **Core Meaning:** "Matayoshi's nunchaku form."
- **Modern Interpretations:** Signature kata within Matayoshi kobudō.
- **Conflicting Ideas & Origins:** Stable eponym (Matayoshi Shinpo/Shinko line).

The title "Matayoshi no Nunchaku" (又吉のヌンチャク) appears simple at first glance, but it carries layered meanings. Literally, it indicates that the form belongs to or is transmitted through the Matayoshi lineage, with the particle "no" (の) serving as a genitive marker, translating to "of." Within the Matayoshi kobudō curriculum, the kata is often referred to simply as "Nunchaku no Kata", where the lineage name acts as an identifier of provenance rather than a formal title. This dual usage illustrates how kata names in Okinawan martial traditions often navigate between function and attribution, anchoring a form either to a location, a person, or, in this case, a family tradition.

The term "nunchaku" (ヌンチャク), written in katakana, suggests that it is a loanword, likely not originally from Japanese or Okinawan vocabularies, and its origins are still debated.

Regardless of its precise etymology, the cultural significance of the name lies in its clarity and directness. Unlike kata named after legendary warriors or specific locations, Matayoshi no Nunchaku reflects the practical spirit of Okinawan kobudō: a straightforward label for a weapon adapted from everyday life. By associating the family name with the form, the kata situates itself within a recognized lineage, while highlighting the transformation of a tool into a weapon. This process defines the Okinawan martial imagination. It pays homage to the ingenuity of past practitioners and serves as a reminder of how necessity shaped the island's martial heritage.

While this understanding of the name offers valuable context, its historical origins reveal the circumstances and individuals that transformed this flexible tool into a formal martial discipline.

Matayoshi no Nunchaku's Historical Roots

The emergence of Matayoshi no Nunchaku underscores the adaptive ingenuity of Okinawan martial culture, complemented by the deliberate preservation efforts of the Matayoshi family. Its status as a formal kata is primarily attributed to the work of Matayoshi Shinko, who systematized many kobudō weapons at a time when traditional practices faced the threat of being overshadowed by modernization and war.

Matayoshi is said to have learned nunchaku from a teacher named Irei, whose instruction emphasized fluidity and leverage. These qualities merged with Matayoshi Shinko's later exposure to Chinese martial arts during his travels in Shanghai and Fuzhou. This synthesis resulted in a kata that was both distinctly Okinawan in spirit and enriched by international influences.

Further efforts in preservation and dissemination were carried out by Shinko's son, Matayoshi Shinpo, who codified the kata within the framework of the Ryukyu Kobudō Federation and later the Zen Okinawa Kobudō Renmei. Under his guidance, Matayoshi no Nunchaku reached a global audience and became a standard component of kobudō training.

The formalization of this kata in the early 20th century addressed both practical and cultural needs. Technically, it provided a structured method for training distance, timing, and coordination with a flexible weapon that requires precision and control. Culturally, it symbolized resistance to the erasure of Okinawan martial identity.

Applying Matayoshi no Nunchaku's Combat Wisdom

At its core, Matayoshi no Nunchaku is not a showcase of flashy techniques or spectacle but rather a deliberate training tool designed to teach the fundamental principles of using a flexible weapon. The kata emphasizes controlled transitions between stances, prioritizing distance, redirection, and angular engagement over the continuous figure-eight movements often associated with widespread nunchaku usage. Strikes are delivered along straight and diagonal lines from the practitioner's four corners, creating a structure that is direct, versatile, and tactically sound.

The body mechanics underlying the form highlight the importance of precision, with wrist articulation, forearm rotation, and rooted footwork working together to harness and redirect the torque generated by the weapon's chain or cord. This foundation teaches practitioners not only to strike effectively but also to remain stable when absorbing or redirecting force.

The kata's distinctive sequence, focusing on two straight strikes followed by two diagonal ones, serves as a technical centerpiece, reinforcing principles of range, unpredictability, and corner-based targeting. Additional components, such as switching the weapon between hands or catching it behind the back, showcase adaptability and control under pressure. These techniques are not just decorative; they are practical skills that allow for recovery from missed strikes or changes in angles during engagement.

More advanced techniques utilize the nunchaku's cord to entangle limbs or other weapons, facilitating disarms, locks, and throws. In bunkai practice, the kata illustrates how a simple flexible weapon can effectively neutralize longer tools through careful timing, trapping, and strategic repositioning.

Matayoshi no Nunchaku stands out due to its strong focus on combative realism. While some martial traditions emphasize performance or spectacle, this form maintains a practical approach designed for close-quarters defense. The kata showcases the versatility of the nunchaku not only as a striking tool but also for trapping, controlling, and unbalancing an opponent. It serves as both a technical guide for using flexible weapons and a living testament to Okinawan ingenuity, where efficiency and adaptability take precedence over flourish, aligning with the principles of the broader Matayoshi system, creating an integrated and coherent approach to kobudō.

The journey of this kata into the broader world can be traced through the preservation efforts of the Matayoshi family and the lineages that carried it beyond Okinawa.

Matayoshi no Nunchaku's Evolving Traditions

The Matayoshi no Nunchaku was first systematized by Matayoshi Shinko and later codified for global dissemination by his son, Matayoshi Shinpo, through the Zen Okinawa Kobudō Renmei. This organization helped spread Okinawan weapon traditions beyond their island origins.

While Matayoshi no Nunchaku remains a kata specific to the Matayoshi lineage, it has gained worldwide popularity through the natural cross-pollination of Okinawan martial arts. Many instructors have trained across multiple systems, and hybrid associations frequently incorporate Matayoshi no Nunchaku into their curricula. Schools affiliated with international Matayoshi organizations, as well as multi-lineage federations, often include this kata to complement their karate instruction, particularly due to its practical combination of striking, trapping, and grappling techniques. Additionally, seminar-based transmission has further expanded its reach, introducing practitioners from diverse styles, including Gensei-ryu and Taira-influenced Ryukyu Kobudō, to the Matayoshi method.

Overall, even when the same kata is practiced across different styles, the techniques and movements can vary significantly due to lineage-specific interpretations. These differences highlight how lineage influences practice, affecting not only the mechanics of the weapon but also the philosophy behind its use.

Matayoshi no Nunchaku's Lasting Impact

Matayoshi no Nunchaku is a remarkable example of Okinawan ingenuity, showcasing how a simple agricultural tool was transformed into a precise weapon embodying discipline. The name itself reflects this practicality: direct, functional, and closely tied to the adaptive spirit of the Matayoshi family. Although it was formally established in the early 20th century under Matayoshi Shinko and his son Shinpo, the kata retains elements of earlier practices, preserving a tradition of flexible weapons that might otherwise have been lost to modernization.

Technically, the form emphasizes angular strikes, distance management, and torque control through grounded stances and coordinated body mechanics. Unlike the more theatrical styles that have popularized the nunchaku in global media, the Matayoshi version is a soberly pragmatic approach. It is reinforced by drills that focus on distance judgment, redirection, and weapon-against-weapon applications. Its strength lies in its practicality; a form designed not for show but for practical self-defense and survival.

While the international dissemination of kata has led to stylistic variations, the core principles of Matayoshi no Nunchaku remain consistent. Today, it is more than just a kata; it acts as a multifaceted bridge between kobudō's agricultural roots and martial sophistication. It reminds practitioners that Okinawan kobudō developed out of necessity and resourcefulness. By studying and preserving this form, martial artists connect with a lineage that honors both cultural heritage and technical refinement.

Maezato no Nunchaku
Okinawa's Preserved Nunchaku Tradition

Introduction to Maezato no Nunchaku

Among the various forms of Okinawan kobudō, few explicitly reveal their authorship as clearly as Maezato no Nunchaku. The term "Maezato" in its title is not merely a village name or a poetic reference; it is the birth surname of Taira Shinken, the 20th-century kobudō reformer born Maezato Shinken in Kumejima. This connection makes the kata a distinct example of a modern composition linked directly to a single individual, thereby contextualizing it within Taira's broader mission to preserve, systematize, and disseminate the traditional weapon arts of Okinawa.

Created in the mid-20th century, Maezato no Nunchaku reflects the urgent cultural preservation efforts of the time. With many old masters passing away and postwar upheaval threatening to erase oral traditions, Taira aimed to codify a representative body of kata for systematic dissemination. By 1955, he had founded the Ryukyu Kobudō Hozon Shinkokai, through which he organized, formalized, and taught a curriculum of weapon forms, including this nunchaku kata, to ensure that Okinawa's martial heritage would endure amidst modernization and globalization.

This chapter examines Maezato no Nunchaku not just as a technical composition but also as a cultural artifact that embodies Taira's preservationist vision. It will explore the implications of its naming, reconstruct its emergence within the context of postwar Okinawa, analyze its combative and pedagogical principles, trace its transmission across lineages, and assess its ongoing significance in the study of kobudō. Through this examination, the discussion will differentiate between verifiable history, oral tradition, and later interpretations, situating the kata within both its historical context and its lasting legacy.

Exploring the Essence of Maezato no Nunchaku

- **Traditional Notation:** 前里のヌンチャク.
- **Script Breakdown:**
  - 前里 (Maezato, surname/toponym);
  - の posessive;
  - ヌンチャク nunchaku.
- **Core Meaning:** "Maezato's nunchaku."
- **Modern Interpretations:** Taira/Matayoshi associated; often demonstrated in Okinawa public demos.
- **Conflicting Ideas & Origins:** Generally consistent.

The title "Maezato no Nunchaku" (前里のヌンチャク) is quite evident in its construction. "Maezato" (前里) refers to the birth surname of Taira Shinken, a modern reformer and preservationist who codified the kata. The particle "no" (の) acts as a possessive marker, translating the title literally to "Maezato's Nunchaku." The final element, "nunchaku" (ヌンチャク), is written in katakana, indicating its status as a relatively modern loanword. The term has ambiguous linguistic roots, often linked to Southern Chinese dialects, such as Min Nan, although no single origin has been definitively established.

In lineages that practice Taira's curriculum, the name has remained consistent, although some English-language sources occasionally refer to it as "Taira no Nunchaku" to emphasize authorship more explicitly. Nonetheless, "Maezato no Nunchaku" is the canonical form listed in kata catalogs and organizational syllabi associated with Taira's Ryukyu Kobudō Hozon Shinkokai.

Culturally, the name "Maezato no Nunchaku" differs from older kata, which often evoke locations, families, or poetic imagery, like "Tsuken Sunakake no Eku" or "Shushi no Kon." By using Taira's birth surname, this title emphasizes its modern origin as a codified form, distinguishing it from traditional kata named after legendary figures, such as Chatan Yara. This reflects the mid-20th-century Okinawan preservationist ethos, as exemplified by Taira Shinken and contemporaries like Matayoshi Shinko, who systematized martial traditions. This likely involved refining existing nunchaku techniques to ensure their survival and transmission to future generations.

Maezato no Nunchaku's Historical Roots

The origins of Maezato no Nunchaku are closely tied to the life and work of Taira Shinken, originally named Maezato Shinken, who was born on Kumejima Island. A veteran of the Japanese army and a lifelong student of martial traditions, Taira trained in karate under Funakoshi Gichin in Tokyo and in kobudō under Yabiku Moden. He dedicated himself to preserving Okinawa's weapon arts.

Beginning in the 1930s, Taira traveled extensively across Okinawa, interviewing elder masters and recording their techniques. His efforts culminated in a catalog of more than forty kata. In 1955, he founded the Ryukyu Kobudō Hozon Shinkokai, the first organization dedicated to safeguarding traditional weapon systems. Through this initiative, he transformed fragmented local practices into a unified curriculum that could be systematically taught both in Okinawa and internationally.

It was within this broader preservation effort that Maezato no Nunchaku was created. Most accounts suggest its development took place in the mid-20th century, around the late 1950s to early 1960s, during a period when Okinawan martial traditions faced the challenges of postwar reconstruction and the opportunities of international expansion. Just as karate was adapted for public education during the early 20th century, kobudō required codified, teachable forms to move beyond insular village transmission. Taira's decision to create a nunchaku kata addressed this need, providing structure where few older precedents existed.

Unlike the bo or sai, which have centuries of documented kata supporting them, the nunchaku did not have a substantial historical corpus. Although the weapon was known, no verifiable pre-20th-century nunchaku kata have been recorded. Therefore, Taira's composition served both a practical and symbolic purpose: it enshrined flexible-weapon principles in a form that could be consistently taught and secured the nunchaku's place alongside other canonical weapons of Okinawan kobudō. In doing so, he ensured that this once marginal implement would become a permanent feature of modern curricula, reflecting the broader adaptive spirit of Okinawan martial culture.

Applying Maezato no Nunchaku's Combat Wisdom

Maezato no Nunchaku reflects Taira Shinken's commitment to functional efficiency instead of ornamental display. The structure of this kata emphasizes angular footwork, compact stances, and controlled swing paths that maintain the weapon on direct, purposeful lines rather than incorporating continuous figure-eight flourishes. Its characteristic rhythm, a cadence of whipping strikes, reversals, and abrupt timing shifts, train practitioners to manage both momentum and distance with precision.

The stances in this kata highlight its distinctive tactical priorities. Variations of kokutsu-dachi and ura-kokutsu-dachi support evasive weight distribution, allowing for quick opening of the hips for defensive transitions and concealed counterattacks. Forward-leaning stances, such as han-zenkutsu-dachi, provide narrow, mobile platforms for advancing strikes while protecting the legs, often with the front foot subtly turned inward for stability during rapid reversals. Transitions into neko-ashi-dachi or more natural, upright positions further emphasize the kata's focus on evasion and adaptability. Unlike the rooted, formal stances found in many karate systems or the grounded power characteristic of Matayoshi's kobudō, Taira's approach prioritizes mobility and compact control, reflecting a practical self-defense orientation.

Movement principles are built on rhythm and flow, where each strike sets up the next. Whipping motions and reversals create continuous momentum, fusing offense and defense. The nunchaku's corded joint enables parries and deflections that transition seamlessly into counters, maintaining momentum with minimal breaks. Footwork ensures control of distance, favoring linear advances, angled retreats, and sudden height shifts to evade while countering. Efficiency is key: attacks are delivered in straight or diagonal lines, close to the body, to reduce exposure and maximize recovery speed.

Technically, the kata develops a versatile range of actions. Core strikes include vertical, horizontal, and diagonal whipping blows, short-arc snaps, and quick reversals aimed at vital targets such as the head, arms, or ribs. The nunchaku's joint is also utilized for wrapping and trapping techniques, intercepting an opponent's limb or weapon to unbalance or disarm them. Bunkai often pairs defensive parries with immediate counters. While some modern interpretations outside of Okinawa embellish the kata with continuous spins for demonstration purposes, the original form emphasizes compact, combat-effective delivery.

Collectively, these principles make Maezato no Nunchaku not merely a flexible-weapon exercise but a practical embodiment of Okinawa's martial ethos, where adaptability, rhythm, and efficiency take precedence over spectacle.

Maezato no Nunchaku's Evolving Traditions

The transmission of Maezato no Nunchaku is closely linked to the institutional framework established by its creator. Through the Ryukyu Kobudō Hozon Shinkokai, Taira provided the organizational platform that introduced the kata from Okinawa to the broader martial arts community. After his death in 1970, the tradition was maintained and expanded by two major successors: Akamine Eisuke, who continued the practice in Okinawa, and Inoue Motokatsu, who promoted it extensively on the Japanese mainland. Senior practitioners like Nakamoto Masahiro have further enhanced the kata's visibility by demonstrating it at events such as the Okinawa Budokan and international gatherings, helping to establish reference standards for its timing and execution.

Despite having relatively modern origins, Maezato no Nunchaku has developed notable stylistic variations across its lineages. In the Ryukyu Kobudō Hozon Shinkokai, the kata remains true to Taira's original form, emphasizing sharp, linear strikes, evasive kokutsu-dachi stances, and rhythmic reversals that seamlessly combine offense and defense. The Shimbukan branch, led by Akamine Eisuke and his successors, retains this foundation but often places greater emphasis on speed and compact stances, resulting in a quicker rhythm suitable for kumite and contemporary training contexts. Inoue Motokatsu's lineage introduced further systematization by dividing the form into Sho and Dai versions, which include grappling applications, joint locks, and defensive responses to knife attacks. This reflects his broader integration of kobudō with the principles of karate.

Other branches preserve the kata with their unique refinements. Tamayose Hidemi's Tesshinkan emphasizes clarity, stability, and efficiency in teaching. At the same time, hybrid karate–kobudō schools often adapt the kata to align it with empty-hand curricula, prioritizing linear strikes over trapping or cord manipulation. Independent lines may retain rustic qualities or locally inspired nuances, with slight variations in rhythm or emphasis that reflect individual interpretation and environmental context.

These variations arise from differences in pedagogy, institutional contexts, and cultural adaptations. Okinawan lineages, such as Taira's Ryukyu Kobudō Hozon Shinkokai and its offshoots, focus on preserving traditional forms rooted in the Ryukyu Kingdom's martial heritage. In contrast, mainland Japanese and international branches adapt the kata to fit structured curricula, competitive demonstrations, or integration with karate. Variations also emerge from linguistic and cultural translations across different teaching environments, as instructors tailor techniques to diverse audiences.

Despite these differences, Maezato no Nunchaku has had a significant impact on the practice of flexible weapons. By anchoring nunchaku training in a codified, combative kata, Taira ensured that it would not devolve into mere acrobatic displays or theatrical performances; instead, it remains grounded in practical principles of distance, timing, and control. Thus, the kata continues to act as both a benchmark of Taira's preservationist efforts and a cornerstone for serious nunchaku instruction worldwide.

Maezato no Nunchaku's Lasting Impact

Maezato no Nunchaku represents a key aspect of Taira Shinken's vision for preserving Okinawan kobudō. Its name, referencing Taira's birth surname Maezato, highlights a focus on authorship and modern standardization rather than on legendary traditions. Unlike many older kata associated with specific places or folklore, this form was developed in the mid-20th century as part of Taira's effort to compile, formalize, and protect Okinawan weapon traditions during a time of rapid modernization and postwar upheaval, which jeopardized their survival.

The kata emphasizes angular precision, efficient rebound control, and the integration of striking, deflection, and trapping into a continuous rhythm. Its compact stances and practical footwork reflect Okinawa's combative realism, teaching timing and distance management with a flexible weapon in a manner that avoids acrobatics or unnecessary ornamentation. This approach provides a systematic introduction to nunchaku principles while reinforcing the broader ethos of kobudō, where the lessons learned from one weapon illuminate those of others.

The form has been widely transmitted through the Ryukyu Kobudō Hozon Shinkokai and its successors, with minor stylistic variations reflecting different pedagogical choices and institutional contexts. Nonetheless, across various lineages, the kata retains its core structure: a teaching framework ensuring that nunchaku practice remains focused on principles rather than performance.

Ultimately, Maezato no Nunchaku is both a product of its time and a safeguard for the future. It exemplifies the deliberate effort to preserve Okinawa's martial heritage in a teachable, standardized form, bridging local creativity with global outreach. As modern practitioners continue to refine the kata, they partake in the same cultural stewardship that characterized Taira's life work; keeping alive not only the techniques of a weapon but also the values of precision, adaptability, and resilience that form the foundation of the Okinawan martial tradition.

SECTION V – KAMA-JUTSU KATA

Okinawa's Sickles: Harvesting Strength and Strategy

The kama, or sickle, is a prime example of how Okinawa transformed agricultural tools into weapons. Originally used for harvesting, the kama features a curved blade and a short handle, making it ideal for martial practice. Techniques involving the kama include lethal slashes and thrusts, along with deceptive traps, hooks, and parries. Practitioners often use paired kama for added versatility. Although bladed weapons were frequently restricted under the Ryukyuan and later Satsuma rule, the kama persevered as both a practical tool and a necessary weapon. In Okinawan martial culture, it embodies adaptability and resourcefulness, teaching practitioners to merge offensive aggression with subtle control. Its presence in kobudō kata emphasizes the balance between everyday life and the demands of self-defense.

HAMA HIGA NO KAMA
Okinawa's Island Reaping Blades

Introduction to Hamahiga no Kama

Few practitioners realize that Hamahiga no Kama is not named after a historical master, but rather derives its identity from Hamahiga Island, a remote outpost of the Ryukyu archipelago steeped in myth. This island is remembered as the home of revered Yukatcha, or scholar-warriors. By invoking this island, the kata situates itself at the intersection of folklore, cultural memory, and martial arts, embodying the uniquely Okinawan tradition of adapting everyday tools into weapons. Practiced with paired kama, or agricultural sickles reimagined for combat, the kata bridges the agrarian and the martial, reflecting both necessity and ingenuity.

Although less widespread than bo, sai, or tonfa kata, Hamahiga no Kama plays a vital role in preserving the agricultural-to-combative lineage within Okinawan kobudō. Its sequences cultivate precision, timing, and control, offering practitioners insight into both the practical application of the weapon and the historical context from which it emerged. The form has been preserved in several traditions, notably within the Ryukyu Kobudō Hozon Shinko Kai and certain schools in the Matsumura Seito Kenshinkan tradition, where it continues to connect modern students with Okinawa's layered past.

This chapter will explore the contested origins of Hamahiga no Kama, tracing its name, geographical associations, and connections to the Pechin class. It will analyze the kata's technical principles and combative logic, examine its transmission across different lineages, and assess its broader cultural and martial significance. In doing so, it aims to position Hamahiga no Kama not only as a weapon form but also as a living repository of Okinawan heritage. To begin this exploration, it is essential first to consider the meaning of the kata's name and the cultural weight carried by its etymology and nomenclature.

Exploring the Essence of Hamahiga no Kama

- **Traditional Notation:** 浜比嘉の鎌. (Hamahiga no Kama)
- **Script Breakdown:**
    - 浜比嘉 Hamahiga (island/family);
    - の posessive;
    - 鎌 "sickle."
- **Core Meaning:** "Hamahiga's kama."
- **Modern Interpretations:** Part of twin-kama curriculum.
- **Conflicting Ideas & Origins:** Stable.

The title Hamahiga no Kama (浜比嘉の鎌) is composed of three elements: Hamahiga (浜比嘉), the name of an island in the Yokatsu archipelago east of Okinawa's main island; the possessive particle no (の), meaning "of"; and kama (鎌), the sickle. Literally translated, the name means "the sickles of Hamahiga." The use of kanji rather than katakana signals that the kata is understood within the context of Okinawa's native geography and cultural heritage, rather than as an imported form.

By invoking Hamahiga, the kata draws upon a site central to Ryukyuan identity. The island is remembered in creation myths as the dwelling place of the progenitors of the Ryukyuan people, and it remained closely tied to Yukatcha (scholar-warrior) traditions during the Ryukyu Kingdom. Naming the kata after Hamahiga thus imbues it with layers of meaning: it evokes not only the practical adaptation of the sickle into a weapon but also a deeper spiritual and cultural lineage, linking practitioners to both the mythic origins and the elite martial heritage of Okinawa.

Hamahiga no Kama's Historical Roots

The precise origins of Hamahiga no Kama are uncertain, much like many Okinawan weapon forms that rely more on oral tradition than written records. Some lineages attribute the kata to a Pechin from Hamahiga Island, linking it either to the 17th-century Higa Peichin or to the later Matsu Higa Peichin of the 19th century. However, the hereditary nature of the Pechin title makes such identifications difficult to confirm, and no surviving documents definitively establish a creator. It is also plausible that the kata emerged as a localized system of kama practice, which was later collected and formalized during the twentieth century. In fact, some scholars suggest that Hamahiga no Kama may represent the codification of older island techniques, brought together in a single structured form by preservationists such as Taira Shinken.

What can be stated with more certainty is when the kata entered the historical record. No pre-modern documentation exists, and the form does not appear in written sources until the mid-twentieth century, when Taira Shinken's landmark text, Ryukyu Kobudō Taikan (1964), included it among the canonical kobudō kata. Its inclusion reflects the broader efforts of that era to safeguard Okinawa's weapon traditions at a time when many were at risk of fading into obscurity. Although its formal appearance in literature is relatively recent, the kata likely preserves much older combative techniques rooted in the agrarian lifestyle of the Ryukyu Islands.

The purpose of Hamahiga no Kama is closely tied to this agricultural context. The kama, a farming sickle, became a natural choice for adaptation as a weapon during periods when conventional arms were restricted, particularly under Satsuma rule. Embedding kama techniques into a kata form allowed practitioners to preserve the methods in a ritualized and repeatable sequence, ensuring transmission even during times of secrecy. Thus, the kata served both practical and cultural functions: it was a method for training precision, timing, and survival skills, as well as a means of safeguarding a distinctly Okinawan martial identity in the face of external control.

Applying Hamahiga no Kama's Combat Wisdom

At its core, Hamahiga no Kama is a study in efficiency and adaptability. It teaches practitioners to manage the lethal potential of the kama while moving with precision, deception, and control. The kata emphasizes the use of paired weapons in complementary roles: one kama parries or traps while the other strikes, creating a constant interplay of offense and defense. This simultaneity reflects the broader Okinawan principle of economy of motion, where every action serves multiple purposes. Notably, the form stresses blade safety, ensuring that all defensive maneuvers are executed on the hardwood shafts rather than the fragile steel edges, which preserves the weapon while maintaining realism.

The stance work provides a structural base for handling these short, curved weapons. Many positions mirror those found in empty-hand karate but are adapted for the kama's size and range, often appearing shorter and more compact than their Japanese counterparts. Zenkutsu dachi (forward stance) serves as the foundation for many advancing techniques, providing forward momentum for slicing strikes or pivoting turns. Heiko dachi (parallel stance) appears at the kata's opening and closing as a neutral readiness posture, with the kama raised and crossed. This symbolizes control and restraint before and after combat. Throughout the kata, the stances remain practical, grounded in balance and mobility, suitable for the close-range, angular combat for which the kama were designed.

The striking methods of Hamahiga no Kama fully utilize the weapon's curved blade and short shaft. Slashing motions form the heart of the kata, delivered in horizontal, vertical, or diagonal arcs that target the ribs, collarbones, or limbs. Thrusting strikes, or tsuki, puncture vital openings with quick, stabbing precision, often accompanied by subtle grip changes that allow the blade to turn upward into the armpit or downward into the abdomen. In some instances, the kama retract along the forearm, transforming the weapon into a reinforced extension of the arm for blunt strikes or grappling counters. This versatility, shifting from lethal cutting to controlling impact, captures the pragmatic adaptability of Okinawan kobudō.

Defensive techniques rely less on hard blocks and more on deflections, traps, and parries, all designed to avoid dangerous blade-to-blade contact. Modified age uke (rising parries) protect the upper body and immediately transition into counterstrikes, while crossing maneuvers use both kama together to ensnare an opponent's weapon. Retracted forearm guards function similarly to ude uke in karate, but with the added reinforcement of the kama shaft, providing both protection and a launching point for counters. These defensive structures are inherently deceptive, often inviting attacks into apparent openings before redirecting them into traps.

Underlying all of this is the kata's sophisticated footwork. Rather than meeting force directly, the practitioner angles off, stepping to the side at a forty-five-degree angle to flank an opponent or retreating while circling the kama overhead to guard the upper line. The form incorporates shifts of height and body level, from rising onto the toes during grip changes to dropping forcefully through the heels for explosive downward strikes. Movements such as nami ashi, a defensive foot lift reminiscent of a wave returning, illustrate how evasive stepping can serve both as a defense against low strikes and a preparation for swift counters. These maneuvers reflect the Ryukyuan preference for body evasion, ensuring safety while setting up decisive retaliation.

In summary, Hamahiga no Kama conveys a philosophy of controlled ferocity. Its techniques train practitioners to manage two short blades with awareness, economy, and respect for their lethality. By combining rooted stances with agile footwork, defensive deception with simultaneous counters, and lethal strikes with non-lethal options, the kata provides a comprehensive education in the use of the kama. Beyond its physical applications, the form fosters mental focus and blade awareness, reminding practitioners that kobudō is not a sport but a means of survival, requiring both technical precision and a profound sense of responsibility.

Hamahiga no Kama's Evolving Traditions

The survival of Hamahiga no Kama, like many forms of kobudō, is largely due to the efforts of twentieth-century preservationists such as Taira Shinken. He systematized numerous weapons kata and ensured their transmission in the postwar era. Thanks to his work and the dedication of committed teacher-student lineages, this form has been passed down through various styles and continues to be practiced today, albeit with notable variations.

As the kata spread beyond its original context, it naturally assumed different expressions based on the tradition. In some schools, it is taught in a compact, pragmatic manner that emphasizes direct techniques suitable for self-defense. In contrast, other schools have rendered it in a more expansive style, featuring fluid transitions and dramatic timing designed for demonstrations and public performances. These differences often arise from lineage-specific training philosophies, the role of kobudō within a given curriculum, or the individual teaching preferences of masters.

Kenwa Mabuni, the founder of Shito-ryu, who was well-versed in kobudō, incorporated weapon training into his system. Many branches of Shito-ryu include Hamahiga no Kama in their kobudō syllabus. Their version employs deeper stances, fluid transitions, and combines influences from Shuri and Naha to provide stability in circular motions. It emphasizes speed and multiple angles, with jabs targeting vital points such as ribs and armpits, angular movements using 45-degree offsets with pivots, and more elaborate turns for fluidity in combinations.

Similarly, some schools in the Kise line of Matsumura Seito Shorin-ryu practice their own rendition of Hamahiga no Kama. They favor natural, upright stances, core-driven downward slashes, and upward jabs. A choked-up grip allows for blunt handle strikes in retracted positions, and defensive techniques include deceptive blocks with the kama positioned along the forearm. They emphasize trapping and quick counters, featuring dynamic shifts with height changes and pivots for flanking, prioritizing unpredictability with a focus on savage, close-range techniques.

The reasons for these variations are manifold. Pedagogical needs often lead to simplification, making complex sequences more accessible to beginners. Conversely, kata adapted for exhibitions tend to prioritize dramatic movements that engage audiences. In karate-dominant schools, the kata may reflect the body mechanics of the host style, whether it be the crisp linearity characteristic of

Shorin-based approaches or the rooted, hip-driven dynamics of Shito-ryu, thus shaping the weapon's expression accordingly.

Although Hamahiga no Kama remains a relatively specialized form, its influence can be seen more broadly. Kama sequences developed in this kata inform the treatment of kama in other hybrid systems, reinforcing essential principles of slashing, trapping, and angular evasion throughout Okinawan kobudō.

Oral traditions function as both cultural narratives and moral teachings. While they may be historically unverified, they sustain the symbolic significance of the kata and remind practitioners that each performance connects to a larger heritage encompassing agrarian life, legend, and martial preservation.

Hamahiga no Kama's Lasting Impact

Hamahiga no Kama serves as both a martial and a cultural artifact, its name connected to the mythic landscape of Hamahiga Island and the traditions of the Ryukyuan Yukatcha. Although its precise origins are uncertain, the kata has been passed down through oral tradition and later codified in the twentieth century, primarily through the preservation efforts of Taira Shinken and his successors.

The technical framework of Hamahiga no Kama showcases the ingenuity of Okinawan kobudō, adapting the farmer's sickle into a versatile weapon capable of simultaneous defense and attack, employing deceptive angles and utilizing the body's core efficiently. Transmission through schools such as Shito-ryu and Matsumura Seito has helped maintain its continuity, even as variations have emerged to meet differing educational goals, performance needs, and stylistic preferences.

Although Hamahiga no Kama is less commonly practiced than more prominent weapons forms, such as those for the sai or tonfa, it retains enduring relevance. It exemplifies the creativity and resilience of Okinawan martial culture, illustrating that kobudō evolved not from battlefield weapons but from everyday tools repurposed for survival. Practicing Hamahiga no Kama today offers both combative training and a cultural connection, preserving not only technique but also the spirit of adaptation and continuity that has shaped Okinawa's martial heritage.

As long as kobudō remains a living tradition, Hamahiga no Kama will continue to link the agrarian past with the martial present. Rooted in island lore and agricultural wisdom, it serves as a reminder that true mastery lies not only in technical precision but also in honoring the history and identity embedded within each form.

KANEGAWA NO NICHOGAMA
Okinawa's Dual Sickle Mastery

Introduction to Kanegawa no Nichogama

Few kata in Okinawan kobudō are as visually striking or as demanding as Kanegawa no Nichogama. This dual-sickle form embodies both artistry and danger through its seamless blend of simultaneous attack and defense. Compared to more commonly practiced weapon forms, such as those for the bo or sai, this kata requires exceptional coordination, timing, and spatial awareness. As a result, it is considered one of the most challenging and sophisticated weapon forms in the kobudō curriculum.

Preserved primarily by the Ryukyu Kobudō Hozon Shinko Kai (Society for the Preservation and Promotion of Ryukyu Kobudō), Kanegawa no Nichogama is not simply a technical exercise but a cultural expression of Okinawan ingenuity. Its execution highlights the unique possibilities of wielding two kama at once: striking, trapping, and parrying across multiple planes in fluid, circular motion.

This chapter explores the kata's complex identity, including its debated origins within the Kanegawa tradition, the advanced principles that underpin its structure, its technical strategies and applications, and the stylistic variations that have emerged across different lineages. In doing so, it positions Kanegawa no Nichogama as both a martial challenge and a living testament to the adaptability and creativity of Okinawan kobudō.

Exploring the Essence of Kanegawa no Nichogama

- **Traditional Notation**: Kanji—鐘川の二丁鎌.
- **Script Breakdown**:

    o 鐘川 Kanegawa - "bell river" or family name (a lineage/teacher).

    o の possessive particle—"of".

    o 二丁鎌 "two [丁] sickles", indicating dual wielding.

- **Core Meaning**: "Kanegawa's Two Sickles"—a kama kata named after a person (Kanegawa Gimu) who specialized in this weapon.
- **Modern Interpretations**: Viewed as a village or family legacy form, reflecting a localized tradition rather than part of standardized system.

The name "Kanegawa no Nichogama" (金川の二丁鎌) consists of three elements: "Kanegawa" (金川), usually interpreted as a geographical or lineage marker; "no" (の), a possessive particle meaning "of"; and "nichogama" (二丁鎌), which literally translates to "two sickles." Written entirely in kanji, the title reflects a localized identity rooted in Okinawan tradition rather than foreign influence, while highlighting the kata's defining feature: the simultaneous use of paired kama.

The exact meaning of "Kanegawa" has been widely debated. Some believe it refers to a specific founder, akin to kata named after figures like Sakugawa or Matsu Higa. However, no historical records confirm the existence of a master by that name, making such attributions speculative at best. Others suggest it might denote a family, a village, or even a lost stylistic label. The most accepted view, particularly within the Ryukyu Kobudō Hozon Shinko Kai, is that "Kanegawa" signifies a codified tradition rather than an individual. According to this interpretation, the kata belongs to a structured curriculum organized by Inoue Motokatsu, the heir to Taira Shinken and the first to receive the Hanshi title under him. Inoue formalized "Kanegawa no Nichogama" in his compendium of Ryukyu Kobudō during the 1970s, along with other "Kanegawa" kata for different weapons, such as the tinbe (shield) and rochin (short spear). In some lineages, both "sho" (lesser) and "dai" (greater) versions of the kata are preserved, reflecting Inoue's systematic approach to organizing the art.

Outside of Inoue's lineage, a few speculative theories persist. Some suggest that "Kanegawa" indicates a stylistic distinction within weapon traditions, emphasizing a unique rhythm, footwork, or fighting principle. Others theorize that the name may originate from an obscure local figure or a misattributed oral tradition that predated Taira Shinken's documentation. However, without written records from the prewar era, these views remain conjectural.

In practice, the name "Kanegawa no Nichogama" serves more as a marker of systematization, linking the kata to the Ryukyu Kobudō canon preserved by Taira Shinken and organized by Inoue Motokatsu. It illustrates how postwar Okinawan martial culture balanced the preservation of oral traditions with the need to formalize curricula for teaching and learning. By categorizing the kata under the "Kanegawa" label, practitioners honor both Okinawa's community-rooted heritage and the modern preservationist efforts that have ensured its survival.

Kanegawa no Nichogama's Historical Roots

Unlike many kobudō kata named after legendary figures, such as Sakugawa or Matsu Higa, Kanegawa no Nichogama does not trace back to a single identifiable master. Instead, it is associated with the work of Inoue Motokatsu (1918–1993), the first student to be awarded the rank of Hanshi by his teacher, Taira Shinken, who founded the Ryukyu Kobudō Hozon Shinko Kai. Inoue played a crucial role in codifying, publishing, and preserving various weapon forms through his multi-volume Ryukyu Kobudō series. Within these texts, he introduced and standardized the Kanegawa series of kata, including the dual-sickle form, thereby securing their place in the modern kobudō canon.

What remains uncertain is whether Kanegawa no Nichogama reflects a preexisting oral tradition that Inoue faithfully recorded, a localized system derived from family or village teachings, or an original synthesis created by Inoue himself, drawing on his extensive knowledge of kama techniques and dual-weapon strategies. No pre-war manuals or archival references have documented the kata, leaving its deeper origins obscured.

The kata entered the written record between 1972 and 1974 with the publication of Inoue's volumes, firmly situating it within the postwar revival of Okinawan kobudō. This was a period of urgency, as masters sought to preserve weapon arts that were threatened by rapid modernization, the legacy of the Satsuma ban on weapons, and the destruction of cultural traditions during World War II. In this context, Kanegawa no Nichogama served both as a technical repository of dual-sickle methods and as part of a broader cultural project aimed at safeguarding and transmitting Okinawa's martial heritage to future generations.

Although its exact origins remain uncertain, the codification of the kata illustrates how postwar masters combined oral tradition, individual creativity, and systematization to preserve Okinawa's weapon traditions during a time when they might have otherwise been lost.

Applying Kanegawa no Nichogama's Combat Wisdom

The challenge of coordinating dual weapons primarily defines Kanegawa no Nichogama. The kata requires practitioners to manage two sickles simultaneously, with each sickle serving distinct roles in offense and defense, often across different planes of motion. This duality exemplifies a hallmark of Okinawan kobudō: the ability to combine adaptability with economy of movement, making every action an opportunity for both protection and counterattack.

The execution of the kata is rooted in circularity and fluid motion. Instead of relying on linear, force-against-force exchanges, techniques generate power through the hips and core, using centrifugal momentum to create slashing arcs, hooking traps, or deflecting parries. The kama's curved blades are designed for such circularity, allowing defenses to flow seamlessly into strikes and redirections. This principle is further emphasized by the kata's focus on dynamic balance, where frequent transitions between rooted stances and single-legged postures test the practitioner's stability and control. Notably, the version practiced at the Ryukyu Kobudō Hozon Shinko Kai headquarters highlights intricate weight shifts, underscoring the sophistication required to wield two blades while maintaining balance.

Technically, the kata incorporates a range of stances, from strong forward and side stances that provide rooted power to compact one-legged positions that facilitate evasive angles and balance management. Striking and blocking often occur simultaneously: one kama parries an incoming blow while the other delivers a slash or thrust in the same motion. This principle of simultaneous offense and defense embodies the efficiency of Okinawan combat strategy. The hooked design of the kama also enables trapping and disarming techniques, allowing practitioners to catch and immobilize an opponent's limb or weapon, followed immediately by a decisive counterattack. Such movements are not only combative but also showcase the strategic versatility of the weapon in close-quarters engagements.

Grip changes further expand the tactical range of the form. Shifting between the standard grip and reverse grip allows the practitioner to adapt seamlessly to different distances and angles, using not only the blade edge but also the wooden shaft or butt of the weapon for striking, blocking, or reinforcing the forearm in defense. This approach encourages practitioners to view the kama as more than just a cutting tool; it becomes a multi-functional extension of the body.

The bunkai, or applied analysis, reveals a kata that excels in the chaos of close-quarters combat. Circular parries transition into angular slashes; hooks disarm or control an adversary while the second weapon strikes; and coordinated dual actions maintain constant pressure on the opponent. The movements also teach control of space through shifting angles, changing levels, and fluid repositioning to manage distance. By combining deception, balance, and multi-directional strikes, Kanegawa no Nichogama embodies the creative ingenuity that defines Okinawan kobudō, transforming an agricultural implement into a refined weapon system while embedding advanced tactical principles into its form.

zanegawa no Nichogama's Evolving Traditions

The preservation of Kanegawa no Nichogama is owed to Inoue Motokatsu's efforts within the Ryukyu Kobudō Hozon Shinko Kai. Like many kata in the modern kobudō canon, its survival reflects a conscious effort to preserve traditions that could have been lost in the postwar era. Today, the kata is most closely associated with lineages that trace back to Taira Shinken and Inoue; however, its execution varies across different schools.

Within Inoue's lineage, the kata is often performed with a "rapid-fire" rhythm, emphasizing continuous flow and smooth transitions, a style that has become widely recognized, even outside of Okinawa. In several branches, Kanegawa no Nichogama is practiced in both sho and dai versions, reflecting a common Okinawan teaching approach where shorter, more compact forms are paired with longer, more expansive versions, striking a balance between efficiency and complexity.

In contrast, the Ryukyu Kobudō Shimbukan, founded by Akamine Eisuke and currently led by his son Hiroshi, preserves a distinct interpretation. Their version emphasizes a more deliberate tempo, incorporating pauses for focused energy and highlighting hip and core power generation, paralleling principles found in Shorin-ryu karate. The application is taught with great attention to practical use, focusing on simultaneous block-and-strike sequences, reverse-grip slashes following deflections, and the significant use of the kama's hook for trapping and disarming. The footwork follows an "H"-shaped embusen and includes one-legged transitions to emphasize balance, marking a subtle but significant divergence from Inoue's faster, fluid approach.

Some schools within the Matsumura Seito Kenshinkan tradition offer yet another perspective, shaped by their lineage from Matsumura Sokon through Soken Hohan and Kise Fusei. This interpretation emphasizes direct and efficient movements with minimal ornamentation, reflecting the school's pragmatic view on combative training. Practitioners focus on simultaneous defense and counterattacks, circular redirections, and shifting body positions to gain a tactical advantage, applying the kama in a straightforward manner for real-world combat rather than for demonstration.

While Kanegawa no Nichogama remains a specialized kata, its dual-sickle mechanics have had a broader influence on kama practice. Principles such as circular defense, coordinated use of paired weapons, and blade trapping are echoed in related kata and drills, reinforcing fundamental lessons across the kobudō curriculum. The diversity of interpretations, ranging from Inoue's rapid continuity to Shimbukan's explosive precision and Kenshinkan's efficient pragmatism, illustrates the vitality of Okinawan martial traditions. Rather than diminishing the kata's identity, these variations affirm its adaptability and the creative resilience of kobudō transmission.

Kanegawa no Nichogama's Lasting Impact

Kanegawa no Nichogama emerges from the modern codification efforts of postwar Okinawa. Named not after an individual master but rather for a set of principles related to weapons combat, it embodies the broader project of systematization led by Taira Shinken and Inoue Motokatsu. The structure of Kanegawa no Nichogama reflects the sophistication of advanced kobudō, featuring fluid balance shifts, adaptable grip work, hip-driven circular motion, and the simultaneous integration of deception, defense, and offense. In this way, it captures both the ingenuity of Okinawan martial arts and the creative resilience involved in their preservation.

Although it is less widely known than the prominent staff or sai kata, Kanegawa no Nichogama holds an essential place in modern kobudō. It maintains the demanding mechanics of dual sickle practice, providing practitioners with a challenge in coordination and timing, as well as a living link to the postwar revival of Okinawa's martial heritage. Studying this kata deepens one's understanding of kama principles more broadly, reinforcing the importance of circular redirection, trapping, and dual-weapon coordination throughout the kobudō curriculum.

As long as Ryukyu Kobudō is practiced, Kanegawa no Nichogama will endure as both a technical challenge and a cultural marker. It is a form that connects the past and present through disciplined practice and careful transmission. Demanding yet rewarding, it stands as a testament to how Okinawan martial traditions transform ordinary tools into extraordinary symbols of resilience, creativity, and identity.

Section VI – Eku-jutsu Kata

Okinawa's Oar: Steering Through Combat

The eku, or boat oar, reflects Okinawa's deep connection with the sea. Used for both fishing and navigation, the eku's broad blade and long shaft were easily adapted for use as a weapon in a maritime culture. Oral traditions describe tactics such as sand-flicking to blind an opponent, showcasing the practical creativity of coastal communities. The techniques involve sweeping strikes, angular leverage, and sudden changes in direction, mirroring both the fluidity of water and the unpredictability of life at sea. As a martial weapon, the eku preserves Okinawa's maritime heritage, symbolizing the integration of livelihood and defense in a culture that depended on both land and sea for survival.

TSUKEN SUNAKAKE NO EKU
Okinawa's Blinding Stroke of the Oar

Introduction to Tsuken Sunakake no Eku

What began as a humble fisherman's oar evolved through necessity and ingenuity into a formidable weapon in Okinawan kobudō. Among the kata found in Okinawan kobudō, Tsuken Sunakake no Eku stands out for its vivid portrayal of coastal life in martial creativity. The name itself evokes the image of a fisherman using his oar to hurl sand and blind or distract an adversary, reminding us that in Okinawa, the boundary between daily survival and martial discipline was often a thin one.

The eku is no ordinary staff. Heavier at the blade end and commonly longer than a standard bo, its design alters balance, timing, and application, making it both awkward and devastating in combat. Originally an essential tool for seafarers, the eku became an improvised weapon when conventional arms were restricted. The kata preserves this transformation: the motions echo rowing, sweeping, and thrusting, refined into tactics of deflection, striking, and destabilization.

Attributed to practices from Tsuken Island, a small islet historically associated with staff traditions, this kata embodies a uniquely maritime aspect of Okinawan kobudō. It serves not only as a record of practical defense but also as a cultural artifact, deeply rooted in the rhythms of island life.

This chapter will explore the contested yet evocative origins of Tsuken Sunakake no Eku, situating it within Okinawa's broader social and historical context. It will analyze the kata's technical and internal principles, trace its transmission and evolution across different lineages, and assess its enduring significance as both a cultural legacy and a living martial practice.

Exploring the Essence of Tsuken Sunakake no Eku

- **Traditional Notation:** 津堅砂掛の櫂
- **Script Breakdown:**
  - 津堅 Tsuken Island.
  - 砂掛 (sunakake) "sand-flicking/throwing."
  - の possessive particle "of".
  - 櫂 (E-kū) indigenous Okinawan term for oar.
- **Core Meaning:** "The Oar of Tsuken That Flicks Sand," alluding to tactics of disrupting an opponent by sand flick, emblematic of island context.
- **Modern Interpretations:** Emphasizes coastal practicality and the clever environmental use of weaponry.
- **Conflicting Ideas & Origins:**

o Naming confusion exists (alternate "Chikin" vs. "Tsuken"), often due to dialect/romanization discrepancies.

o Broadly accepted origin as a local Tsuken kata; no significant controversy.

The name "Tsuken Sunakake no Eku" (津堅砂掛けの櫂) intricately combines elements of geography, technique, and tool, reflecting Okinawa's maritime culture. "Tsuken" (津堅) refers to Tsuken Island, a small islet off Okinawa's eastern coast that is closely associated with multiple staff traditions. Like other kata named after locations, this title likely indicates either the kata's origin or its significance within the local fishing communities.

The term "sunakake" (砂掛け) translates to "sand-flinging" or "sand-scattering," which refers to the distinctive technique of using the oar's flat blade to scoop and throw sand into an opponent's eyes. This clever tactic serves as an environment-specific defense, showcasing the ingenuity of Okinawan combat methods. The particle "no" (の) acts as a possessive, connecting the various elements, while "eku" (櫂) denotes the oar itself.

In Uchinaaguchi, the Okinawan language, the word is pronounced closer to "ueeku" and directly refers to the boat oar that was essential for seafaring and fishing. The weaponized eku differs significantly from the bo: its heavier blade end alters balance and timing, and its broader surface allows for sweeping strikes and the distinctive sand-flicking maneuver.

Linguistic variations add another layer of complexity. In some sources, the kata is referred to as "Tsuken Sunakake no Kon," reflecting the overlap between eku and staff practice, or as "Chikin Sunakake no Eku," an alternate name influenced by dialectal shifts and oral traditions. Additionally, there is a possible historical connection to Tsuken Akachu ("the Red Man of Tsuken"), a semi-legendary figure linked to eku kata, suggesting that the name preserves both a geographic and personal legacy.

Beyond linguistic aspects, the name carries significant cultural meaning. By associating the kata with Tsuken Island and the imagery of flicking sand, it highlights the connection between daily livelihood and self-defense in Okinawan kobudō. What was once an essential tool for fishermen has evolved into a weapon of necessity, a transformation represented in kata that honors both creativity and survival. Thus, the name encapsulates not only technical detail but also the essence of Okinawa's seafaring identity, where environment and combat are inextricably linked.

Tsuken Sunakake no Eku's Historical Roots

The roots of Tsuken Sunakake no Eku can be traced back to the fishing community of Tsuken Island (Chikin-jima), where local oral traditions connect the kata to both significant figures and maritime life. Legends tell of a fisherman named Akachu, who received his nickname due to his sun-darkened skin. He learned staff techniques from Chikin Uekata Masanori, a defeated nobleman who sought refuge on the island. Akachu adapted these teachings for use with the oar, creating the distinctive sand-flicking maneuver designed to blind or distract opponents in coastal combat. Whether these stories are understood as literal or symbolic, they illustrate a culture where survival hinged on the resourceful use of everyday tools.

However, the form practiced today cannot be solely traced back to these legends. The kata was first documented in the 20th century, during a time when Okinawan kobudō was being systematically preserved. Two key figures played crucial roles in this preservation. Matayoshi Shinko and his son Matayoshi Shinpo incorporated the eku into their family's kobudō tradition, naming it Chikin Akachu no Eku Di and explicitly connecting it to the legendary figures of Tsuken. At the same time, Taira Shinken, the leading authority on codifying Ryukyu kobudō, recorded and systematized the form, securing its place within the curriculum of the Ryukyu Kobudō Hozon Shinkokai.

These two preservation efforts have resulted in the kata existing in two distinct lineages: the Matayoshi tradition, which is grounded in folklore and oral heritage, and the Taira tradition, which is based on modern codification. Each lineage emphasizes different aspects, but together they show how the fishing culture of Tsuken Island has been enshrined in the broader martial canon of Okinawa.

Applying Tsuken Sunakake no Eku's Combat Wisdom

The Tsuken Sunakake no Eku highlights the transformation of a fisherman's oar into a versatile and deceptive weapon. Its fundamental principles are shared across different lineages but are expressed uniquely depending on their transmission.

At the core is the sunakake technique, known as the iconic sand flick. By dragging or scooping the paddle through sand and flinging it toward an opponent's face, the practitioner demonstrates both environmental awareness and psychological disruption. This reflects the pragmatic approach of Okinawan martial arts: combat is not solely about power; it also involves seizing advantages through cleverness.

The design of the eku, which is heavier at one end, requires techniques based on rotation, whipping force, and leverage. Circular strikes and sweeping motions mimic rowing, while thrusts with the butt or blade edge target vital points. Parrying actions redirect force and often blend smoothly into counterattacks; a block can transition into a strike, or a sweep can destabilize an opponent before a thrust. Footwork is agile and evasive, characterized by angled steps and sliding entries that maintain balance while maximizing reach.

The distinctions among lineages are crucial. The Matayoshi version emphasizes grounded stances, practical bunkai (application of techniques), and, in some interpretations, small functional jumps for surprise and reorientation. These movements enhance unpredictability, reminiscent of the island folklore regarding sudden sand-flick tactics on the beach. In contrast, the Taira Shinken version does not incorporate jumps. Instead, it focuses on a whipping back-and-forth motion that allows practitioners to strike, recover, and reverse the eku in a continuous cycle. This method creates an unbroken rhythm where offense and defense merge fluidly, embodying Taira's preservationist emphasis on efficiency and flow.

Together, these interpretations illustrate the adaptability of the eku. One lineage highlights grounded realism and dramatic tactical flourishes, while the other distills the weapon into a study of momentum, rhythm, and rapid adaptability.

Tsuken Sunakake no Eku's Evolving Traditions

The modern transmission of Tsuken Sunakake no Eku illustrates the combined efforts of Matayoshi Shinko and Taira Shinken, whose students adapted the form within various organizational contexts.

Within the Matayoshi lineage, the kata is preserved as Chikin Akachu no Eku Di, a name that honors Tsuken Island and the fisherman Akachu. This version emphasizes strong stances, practical bunkai, and the iconic sand-flick, often accompanied by small jumps that add an element of tactical deception. It is practiced not only in the Matayoshi family's Kodokan dojo but also in related organizations, including the Kenshinkan system of Matsumura Seito, where it is performed without jumps while still retaining the same grounded mechanics and island-linked heritage.

In contrast, the Taira lineage preserved within the Ryukyu Kobudō Hozon Shinkōkai interprets the form quite differently. Taira's version eliminates jumps altogether, opting instead for a reciprocal whipping motion in which each strike prepares for the next reversal of the eku. This creates a distinctive rhythm and aesthetic, prioritizing continuous flow and rapid adaptation over dramatic shifts. Successors like Akamine Eisuke and his son Hiroshi at the Ryukyu Kobudō Shimbukan have maintained this emphasis, producing a version known for its crisp execution and clarity of form. Further offshoots, such as the Tesshinkan under Tamayose Hidemi, reflect this Taira-derived lineage while adding subtle refinements.

Meanwhile, the Tsuken Kobudō Hozon Kai, associated with practitioners native to Tsuken Island, preserves a less formalized version sometimes referred to as Tsuken Sunakake no Ueku-di. Notable performers such as Nakamoto Masahiro demonstrate this style, showcasing its rustic qualities and shedding light on local traditions that may predate systematization.

These variations are not contradictions but rather exemplify the vitality of kobudō as a living tradition. The Matayoshi line emphasizes folklore and functional realism, the Taira line stresses fluid continuity and preservation, and local island traditions sustain a sense of place. Together, they ensure that Tsuken Sunakake no Eku survives not as a static artifact but as a multifaceted expression of Okinawa's maritime heritage and martial resilience.

Tsuken Sunakake no Eku's Lasting Impact

Tsuken Sunakake no Eku is more than just a record of oar-fighting; it serves as a living chronicle of Okinawa's ingenuity, where everyday tools became weapons, and survival sparked creativity. Its name is closely linked to Tsuken Island and reflects the maritime identity of its people. The defining sand-flicking technique exemplifies the practical application of the environment in combat.

Legends of figures such as Chikin Uekata Masanori and Akachu enhance the kata's cultural significance, even though they are primarily rooted in oral tradition rather than verified records.

The kata's true endurance lies in how it was preserved and shaped by 20th-century masters. Through the Matayoshi lineage, it has been passed down as Chikin Akachu no Eku Di, rooted in folklore and practiced with strong stances, practical bunkai, and, in some versions, small jumps that emphasize its deceptive tactics.

In contrast, the Taira Shinken lineage has developed a strikingly different interpretation: a form without jumps that focuses on back-and-forth momentum, allowing offense and defense to flow seamlessly in rapid succession. Subsequent traditions, such as Kenshinkan, Shimbukan, and Tesshinkan, continue to refine these different expressions, while the Tsuken Kobudō Hozon Kai preserves more rustic island interpretations.

Together, these strands of transmission illustrate not contradiction but continuity through diversity. Each version safeguards distinct aspects of Okinawa's maritime heritage: Matayoshi's connection to legend and local color, Taira's emphasis on systemization and fluidity, and the islanders' preservation of a less formalized practice.

Today, Tsuken Sunakake no Eku remains a challenging study of adaptability, balance, and environmental awareness. It reminds practitioners that kobudō is not only about mastering weapons but also about carrying forward cultural identity through movement. By training in this kata, modern students inherit both a rigorous technical discipline and a living link to Okinawa's coastal past. Its survival across various lineages ensures that, whether performed with grounded power or fluid rhythm, the kata continues to embody the resilience and creativity that define the Ryukyuan martial spirit.

SECTION VII – TEKKO-JUTSU KATA

Okinawa's Iron Knuckles: The Hidden Fist of Force

The tekko is a fist-loading weapon that resembles brass knuckles. It is often made from paired horseshoes or an iron bar, with a bent strap, that resembles a metal stirrup, embodying the Okinawan martial arts ethos of adaptation. Compact and easily concealed, tekko enhance the power of punches while also allowing for trapping and blocking techniques. Their origins likely stem from repurposed horse tack or ironwork, which were gradually refined into specialized weapons within the kobudō tradition.

Although tekko may not be as visually striking as larger weapons, they reflect a culture of practical ingenuity; taking available materials and transforming them into tools for protection. In Ryukyuan martial culture, tekko kata preserve the principles of efficiency, close-range power, and the seamless integration of weapons with empty-hand techniques.

MAEZATO NO TEKKO
Okinawa's Iron Knuckle Legacy

Introduction to Maezato no Tekko

Few Okinawan weapon kata capture the ingenuity of the Ryukyuan martial tradition as vividly as Maezato no Tekko. This form embodies the remarkable resourcefulness of Okinawan practitioners, who transformed ordinary objects into compact handheld weapons. Known as tekko, these "fist-loads" could enhance the power of a punch, protect the knuckles, and turn basic strikes into decisive defenses at close range. This adaptation seamlessly extends the principles of empty-hand karate into a weaponized form, requiring little adjustment while offering significant effectiveness. It reflects one of the central themes of Okinawan kobudō: the transformation of everyday tools into instruments of survival under restrictive social and political conditions.

Maezato no Tekko was codified in the 20th century by Taira Shinken, originally named Maezato Shinken, whose preservationist vision safeguarded many endangered weapon traditions. Within his organization, Ryukyu Kobudō Hozon Shinkukai, the tekko kata exemplifies both simplicity and sophistication; its mass reinforces fundamental strikes while also allowing for trapping, blocking, and joint manipulation.

This chapter will explore the kata's historical origins, its etymology and cultural associations, the combative principles encoded in its sequences, and its transmission through Taira's lineage and beyond. In doing so, it situates Maezato no Tekko not merely as a technical exercise but as part of a larger narrative of Okinawan resilience and creativity, where even the name itself reveals a story of personal authorship, cultural identity, and the reimagining of humble tools into weapons of survival.

Exploring the Essence of Maezato no Tekko

- **Traditional Notation:** 前里の鉄甲.
- **Script Breakdown:**

    o 前里 (Maezato): Taira Shinken's birth surname—Maezato.

    o の possessive particle—"of".

    o 鉄甲 **(**tekko): "iron armor" or "iron knuckle"—a fist-loading weapon.

- **Core Meaning:** "Maezato's Iron Knuckles"
- **Modern Interpretations:** The association with Maezato signifies formal authorship and codification in Ryūkyū kobudō by Taira Shinken.
- **Conflicting Ideas & Origins:** Virtually no debate; widely recognized as one of Taira's personally authored kata.

The title "Maezato no Tekko" (前里の鉄甲) is both clear and revealing. The first part, "Maezato" (前里), is the birth surname of Taira Shinken, a prominent preservationist of Okinawan kobudō. By using his family name, this kata asserts its authorship and lineage, setting it apart from older forms that are named after regions, legendary figures, or poetic images. The second part, the particle "no" (の), serves as a possessive connector, while "tekko" (鉄甲) literally means "iron armor." In practice, this term refers to the fist-loading weapon, often adapted from stirrups, horseshoes, or forged iron pieces, which is used to enhance the striking power of the hand. Unlike some weapon names that are rendered in katakana to suggest foreign influence, "tekko" is written in kanji, emphasizing its deep-rootedness in Okinawan martial vocabulary.

In contrast to many older kata whose origins are obscured by oral tradition, the name Maezato no Tekko is unambiguous. Reputable sources from the Ryukyu Kobudō Hozon Shinkokai and related lineages consistently list this kata under the same name, with little variation. This clarity stands in sharp contrast to the vague or absent titles found in earlier eras, where the use of tekko was practical but rarely formalized within kata.

The name preserves the identity of Taira Shinken, born Maezato, as both an innovator and a custodian of tradition. It also specifies the weapon central to this form. In doing so, the title situates the kata firmly within the mid-20th-century movement of codification, indicating a conscious effort at preservation and systematization rather than an ancient village tradition. Therefore, studying Maezato no Tekko allows one to engage directly with Taira's legacy, highlighting the intersection of personal authorship and cultural continuity in the naming of this form.

Understanding the clarity and intent behind its name lays the foundation for exploring the context of its creation, during which Taira Shinken transformed tekko practice into a formalized kata at a critical time for the preservation of Okinawan martial arts.

Maezato no Tekko's Historical Roots

The origins of Maezato no Tekko can be traced back to the mid-20th century, when Taira Shinken dedicated his life to preserving Okinawan weapon traditions. In the wake of World War II, many kata were at risk of disappearing, prompting Taira to codify more than forty forms from various lineages. In some instances, he composed kata himself to address gaps in the curriculum. Maezato no Tekko falls into this latter category; it was created to ensure that the fist-load weapon was included in the emerging canon of Ryukyu kobudō.

The systematization of this form occurred in the 1950s and 1960s, during a time when Taira was actively organizing the Ryukyu Kobudō Hozon Shinkokai. This postwar period was marked by a concerted effort to protect Okinawan cultural practices, including martial arts. By formalizing the tekko into a structured kata, Taira ensured that this weapon would be taught within a coherent system, rather than be left to fragmentary local practices.

The motivation behind this codification was both practical and symbolic. The tekko, a simple fist-loading implement, exemplified the Okinawan tradition of transforming everyday tools into effective self-defense instruments. While popular accounts often depict it as a weapon used by farmers or fishermen made from horseshoes or stirrups, historical evidence suggests that such weapons were more likely to have been maintained by members of the Yukatchu class. Regardless, Taira's decision to include the tekko in his curriculum reinforced the identity of kobudō as a repository of adaptive ingenuity, where humble tools became formalized methods of combat.

In this context, Maezato no Tekko represents both continuity and innovation. It embodies centuries of Okinawan creativity in weapon design while also being a distinctly modern creation that showcases Taira's influence in shaping the kobudō tradition to ensure its survival in a rapidly changing world.

Applying Maezato no Tekko's Combat Wisdom

Maezato no Tekko combines the principles of Okinawan kobudō with the close-quarters framework of Karate, where simplicity is enhanced by precision. Unlike longer weapons, the tekko requires angular movements, stable stances, and tight control, prioritizing small actions that lead to significant results. This form emphasizes economy of motion through short strikes, sharp redirections, and subtle evasions that reflect the mechanics of empty-hand kata, while being enhanced by the added weight of the weapon.

The kata favors stances such as zenkutsu dachi for rooted strikes, neko-ashi-dachi for mobility and evasion, and kokutsu-dachi for defensive redirection. Each stance is practical rather than decorative, allowing the practitioner to generate power from the hips while maintaining the agility to respond to multiple opponents. The posture remains upright and centered, ensuring that the additional weight of the tekko enhances strikes without compromising balance. At the same time, the rhythm alternates between deliberate defenses and explosive counters, mimicking the unpredictable nature of real combat.

Force is generated through the entire kinetic chain, from the floor, through the hips, and into the shoulders, rather than relying solely on arm strength. As a result, the tekko serves as a weight multiplier, transforming basic punches into powerful, percussive blows. Breathing is synchronized with impact, alternating relaxation with sharp focus to stabilize each strike and prevent energy loss. The kata incorporates straight punches reinforced by the metal body of the tekko, circular hooks for intercepting or unbalancing an opponent, and trapping techniques that immobilize joints or redirect an opponent's weapon. The applications focus on combinations of short, targeted strikes delivered in rapid succession, rather than sweeping motions, often highlighting grappling-style techniques. Defensive strategies emphasize redirection and blocking, combined with sharp pivots and 180-degree turns reminiscent of classical karate kata like Jion, allowing the practitioner to counter threats from multiple directions.

In summary, Maezato no Tekko is a study in concentrated force and practical efficiency. It exemplifies the Okinawan philosophy of transforming simple tools into highly adaptable weapons, training practitioners to seamlessly merge stability, precision, and adaptability in close-range encounters.

Maezato no Tekko's Evolving Traditions

Since its codification by Taira Shinken, Maezato no Tekko has remained closely connected to the institutions and senior disciples dedicated to preserving his mission. In Okinawa, the kata has been maintained through the Ryukyu Kobudō Hozon Shinkokai, the organization that Taira himself founded. It serves as a representative fist-load form within their curriculum. Following Taira's passing in 1970, the transmission of the kata occurred through two main channels: Akamine Eisuke, who took over leadership in Okinawa, and Inoue Motokatsu, who established the Ryukyu Kobujutsu system in mainland Japan. Both individuals ensured the kata's survival, though their teaching styles differed, reflecting their unique approaches to kobudō instruction.

From these origins, Maezato no Tekko spread into related organizations. The Ryukyu Kobudō Tesshinkan, founded by Tamayose Hidemi (a student of Akamine), retains the kata and requires demonstrations of bunkai as part of rank examinations, highlighting its role as both a practical and formal exercise. The Shimbukan, also descended from Akamine, teaches the form with slight refinements, such as adjustments to the embusen for consistency in presentation. Additionally, the kata is practiced in Shorin-ryu Matsumura Seito Kenshinkan, where the principles are interpreted through the system's characteristic upright and natural postures, enhancing agility in close-quarters combat. This interpretation enhances agility in close-quarters combat. It reflects the historical emphasis of Shuri-te on practical self-defense against armed or multiple attackers, focusing on precise and timed entries using techniques that accelerate like a whip. The approach avoids overcommitment, emphasizes evasion, and integrates defense and offense, creating a unique rhythm within Taira's original composition.

The stylistic variations between these branches are modest yet significant. Some organizations emphasize different strike angles or modify footwork transitions, while interpretations of bunkai can vary from blunt, percussive techniques to more joint-manipulative or trapping applications. Even seemingly minor details, such as whether a tekko block lands with the iron cross-bar against the wrist or with the ball at the side, illustrate the diversity of interpretation across lineages. These variations do not diminish the kata's integrity; instead, they showcase the adaptability of a form designed to be less of a rigid template and more of a vessel for the core principles of close-quarters combat.

Maezato no Tekko's Lasting Impact

Maezato no Tekko is a prime example of how modern kobudō codification has helped preserve endangered weapon practices. The name of the form links it directly to its creator, Taira Shinken (originally Maezato Shinken), who codified the compact fist-load weapons form, enhancing ordinary punches into powerful close-quarter strikes. Systematized in the mid-20th century, this kata reflects Taira's broader effort to preserve Okinawan martial traditions at a time when they were at risk of disappearing due to war and modernization.

Technically, the form emphasizes efficiency and practicality through short, angular footwork, compact stances, and the enhanced striking power provided by the tekko's added weight. Its applications focus on blunt effectiveness, such as intercepting attacks, targeting joints, and delivering concentrated blows. Although minor refinements have been made over time by different lineages, the essence of the kata has remained consistent, solidifying its position as a cornerstone of the tekko curriculum within kobudō systems worldwide.

Beyond its combative aspects, the kata holds significant symbolic meaning. It demonstrates Okinawa's ability to adapt everyday tools into disciplined martial traditions, reclaiming cultural heritage under challenging historical circumstances. Practicing Maezato no Tekko enables practitioners not only to gain technical knowledge but also to assume the responsibility of cultural stewardship, preserving a form that embodies Okinawan resilience and creativity. Ultimately, Maezato no Tekko is more than just a kata; it serves as a bridge between Okinawa's past and present, continuing the legacy of a culture that transformed necessity into lasting art.

KAKAZU NO TEKKO

Okinawa's Modern Legacy of the Tekko

Introduction to Kakazu no Tekko

Unlike many weapon forms from Okinawa, whose origins are often shrouded in oral tradition, Kakazu no Tekko stands out for bearing the name of its acknowledged creator, Mitsuo Kakazu. As a postwar kobudō instructor within the Matayoshi lineage, Kakazu formalized this kata to capture the compact and forceful logic of the tekko. He ensured that the more prominent weapons, such as the bo and sai, would not overshadow the unique applications of the tekko. His efforts provided the humble fist-load tool turned weapon with a structured method for preservation. In this way, Kakazu no Tekko represents both local innovation and the broader mid-20th-century revival of Okinawa's martial heritage.

The tekko is a small yet powerful weapon, appreciated for its ability to enhance strikes, trap or redirect an opponent's limbs, and provide defensive reinforcement in close-quarter combat. Kakazu no Tekko is included in modern curricula associated with Matayoshi kobudō, as well as Okinawa Kenpo and other kobudō lineages linked to Odo Seikichi, where it is sometimes referred to as "Odo no Tekkos Ni (Kakazu no Tekko)." This cross-labeling highlights the fluidity of postwar transmission, as kata were preserved, renamed, and adapted within parallel traditions during the period of renewed systematization.

This chapter explores the etymology and cultural significance of the kata's name, investigates competing claims regarding its origin and attribution, analyzes the technical logic of its sequences, and traces its evolution across different lineages. In doing so, it positions Kakazu no Tekko not just as a modern addition to the kobudō canon but also as a testament to Okinawa's enduring martial creativity and adaptability.

Exploring the Essence of Kakazu no Tekko

- **Traditional Notation**: 嘉数の手甲 or 鉄甲
- **Script Breakdown**:

    o 嘉数 (Kakazu): Okinawan surname/place.

    o の possessive particle—"of".

    o 手甲 (tekko): hand guard; alternately 鉄甲: iron guard, weapon.

- **Core Meaning**: "Kakazu's Iron Knuckles"—a tekko kata named for its creator, Kakazu Mitsuo.

- **Modern Interpretations**: Highlights personal lineage; uncontroversial in attributed authorship.

- **Conflicting Ideas & Origins**:

- Connection with Kakazu Mitsuo is accepted in Matayoshi and Odo lineages.
- Minimal dispute exists; the form is consistently attributed to that individual in modern lineages.

The title Kakazu no Tekko (嘉数の手甲 / 嘉数の鉄甲) reflects both personal authorship and the weapon's distinctive identity. "Kakazu" is an Okinawan surname, here honoring Mitsuo Kakazu, the kata's acknowledged creator. The particle no (の) serves as a possessive marker, while tekko is written in two common forms: 手甲, meaning "hand guard" or gauntlet, and 鉄甲, literally "iron armor" or "iron fist." The coexistence of these kanji underscores the tekko's dual nature as both a protective hand-guard and a fist-loaded striking tool. Unlike other weapons such as the nunchaku, whose name is usually rendered in katakana, tekko remains consistently written in kanji, signaling its status as a native term within the Japanese-Okinawan lexicon.

While there is little dispute about the name itself, variations do exist across lineages. In Odo Seikichi's Okinawa Kenpo/Kobudō, the kata appears as Odo no Tekkos Ni ("Odo's Tekko No. 2"), a renaming that reflects curricular adaptation rather than a contested origin.

Culturally, naming the kata after Kakazu situates it within a postwar trend of explicitly linking forms to their teachers, part of a broader effort to preserve and standardize kobudō under conditions of cultural upheaval. Just as Maezato no Tekko immortalized Taira Shinken's birth surname, Kakazu no Tekko affirms the authorial role of Mitsuo Kakazu. It honors not only the individual who systematized the form, but also the spirit of resilience in Okinawan martial culture—where ordinary tools became weapons, and weapons became traditions fit for transmission to future generations. In this sense, the name embodies both personal innovation and collective preservation, anchoring the kata firmly within Okinawa's martial renaissance of the mid-20th century.

Kakazu no Tekko's Historical Roots

Kakazu no Tekko is notable among kobudō kata for its clear authorship, distinctly attributed to Mitsuo Kakazu (嘉数 光男). He was a postwar kobudō practitioner who trained directly under Matayoshi Shinko (又吉眞光, 1888–1947), one of Okinawa's most celebrated custodians of weapon traditions. After Shinko's death, Kakazu furthered his studies with Shinko's son, Matayoshi Shinpō (又吉眞豊, 1921–1997), ensuring that his practice remained rooted within the Matayoshi lineage.

This kata was created in the mid-20th century, during a time of cultural reconstruction in Okinawa following the devastation of World War II. During this period, prominent figures such as the Matayoshi family worked to codify and expand kobudō curricula, thereby safeguarding endangered traditions and structuring them for both Okinawan and international students. Kakazu's development of a dedicated tekko kata aligned with this movement, elevating the weapon from a mere supplementary training tool to a formally recognized form worthy of preservation.

The design of the kata reflects the significant influence of Matayoshi Shinko's extensive studies in China, where he trained in Fujian and Shanghai martial traditions that focused on compact, short-range weapons and integrated striking techniques with trapping, joint control, and angular evasion. Kakazu no Tekko embodies this legacy, showcasing the tekko not only as a fist-load enhancer for strikes but also as a tool for hooking, redirecting, and controlling an opponent in close-quarters combat. By distilling these principles into a kata, Kakazu made the tekko accessible for structured practice, grading, and transmission through a repeatable sequence.

Though tekko are believed to be derived from practical tools such as stirrups, net-hauling grips, or iron implements, there are no documented premodern kata specifically for the weapon. Thus, Kakazu no Tekko represents an innovation rather than the preservation of a lost prototype. Its angles, short-arc power generation, and logic of close-quarters combat resonate with broader Okinawan combat principles, as well as the adaptability emphasized by Shinko, which was influenced by Chinese martial arts. In this respect, Kakazu's kata serves not only as a personal contribution but also as a living reflection of the Matayoshi family's synthesis of Okinawan and Chinese martial traditions, woven into the broader postwar effort to preserve Okinawa's cultural heritage.

Applying Kakazu no Tekko's Combat Wisdom

Kakazu no Tekko embodies the principles of close-range combat, emphasizing stability, efficiency of movement, and precise control over flashy displays. The kata utilizes narrow, upright stances typical of the Matayoshi tradition, such as a modified kiba-dachi for stability and a neko-ashi-dachi for evasive mobility. These stances enable practitioners to quickly move in and out of range, employing half-steps and angled entries to navigate distances against opponents wielding longer weapons. Power is generated not through exaggerated movements but through compact hip rotation and grounding the body, allowing energy to transfer smoothly from the ground into the fist. This method, influenced by Chinese quanfa through Matayoshi Shinko, produces strikes that are both powerful and whip-like without compromising balance.

The mass of the tekko naturally enhances basic punches, but the kata offers much more than raw impact. Its sequences emphasize reinforced thrusting punches for penetrating power, slashing techniques using the edges of the tekko, and short, snapping strikes aimed at vital targets such as the jawline, temple, or ribs. Defensive techniques include hooking blocks, which not only intercept attacks but also trap limbs or seize weapon shafts, allowing for effective counters. From these positions, practitioners can push, twist, or lock joints, blending empty-hand techniques with weapon dynamics. This technical logic mirrors empty-hand kata such as Seisan, where compact stances, angular entries, and decisive bursts of power also reflect control in close quarters and efficient redirection of force.

The kata's rhythm reinforces these principles. Movements alternate between deliberate defensive positions and quick offensive bursts, with breathing coordinated to tighten upon impact and relax between strikes. This relaxed–tense dynamic helps control rebound effects, prevent over-rotation, and maintain readiness for continuous exchanges. Concepts such as muchimi and kakei guide transitions, allowing the tekko to serve not only as a striking tool but also as an instrument for redirection and dominance in close-quarters combat.

In this way, Kakazu no Tekko exemplifies the practical ethos of Okinawan kobudō: it is compact, efficient, and deeply integrated with the body mechanics of karate while being refined by fluid adaptability derived from Chinese influences. Similar to its empty-hand counterpart Seisan, it showcases how Okinawan martial culture continuously adapted a core set of principles across both weapon and unarmed traditions.

Kakazu no Tekko's Evolving Traditions

Kakazu no Tekko was created and transmitted by Kakazu Mitsuo, who codified the kata within the framework of Matayoshi kobudō and taught it directly to his students. Among these students was Odo Seikichi, the founder of the Okinawa Kenpo Karate Kobudō Association. Odo's adoption of the form ensured its spread beyond the Matayoshi circle. In Odo's system, the kata is often referred to as Odo no Tekko Ni, with an explicit note stating it is "also known as Kakazu no Tekko." This renaming honors both the kata's origin and its transmission through Odo's teachings. This dual labeling illustrates how postwar Okinawan martial culture balanced fidelity to the original form with adaptations for institutional or pedagogical purposes.

The stylistic differences between lineages are modest yet highlight Okinawa's broader pattern of kata variation. Some schools alter the embusen by shifting angles or refining transitions, while others change the rhythm or tempo for clarity in instruction or demonstration. These adjustments are not radical changes but rather slight inflections shaped by the context of each dojo. In Matayoshi-line schools, the bunkai typically emphasizes fluid counters to grabs and weapon attacks, with movements that flow seamlessly from parrying to seizing to striking. In contrast, Odo-line practice often focuses on linear efficiency, illustrating the kata's suitability for defending against multiple opponents and enhancing its relevance for modern self-defense training.

The reasons for these divergences stem from practical considerations. Factors such as dojo space, teaching methods, and performance contexts lead to slight alterations in footwork and linking movements. Additionally, the institutional framework plays a role; for example, Odo's federation designated the kata as Tekko Ichi and Ni in their instructional materials, reinforcing sequencing choices that differ from Matayoshi's curriculum. Despite these differences, the fundamental principles of Kakazu no Tekko, compact, percussive striking, precise limb control, and effective counterattacks, remain consistent across lineages. The variations should not be viewed as contradictions but as evidence of a living tradition capable of preserving Kakazu's original intent while adapting to diverse teaching environments.

Kakazu no Tekko's Lasting Impact

Kakazu no Tekko is one of the few kobudō kata with a clear line of authorship, named in honor of Mitsuo Kakazu. The weapon is identified by the characters 手甲 ("hand guard" or gauntlet) and 鉄甲 ("iron fist"), which are both found in contemporary sources. This highlights the dual identity of the tekko as both a protective device and a fist-loading weapon. Unlike Taira Shinken's established Maezato no Tekko, Kakazu no Tekko emerged around the same time through the networks of Matayoshi kobudō and Odo Seikichi's Okinawa Kenpo Karate Kobudō Association. It provided a structured framework for a weapon that was often limited to drills rather than formal kata.

Technically, the form captures the combative essence of the tekko, featuring compact stances, angular footwork, snapping percussive strikes, and the integration of trapping and framing motions suitable for close-quarters encounters. The principles of Kakazu no Tekko echo those found in tekko kihon and even in empty-hand kata such as Seisan, demonstrating how Okinawan martial philosophy intertwines weapons and unarmed techniques under a shared tactical approach. While there are minor stylistic differences between the Matayoshi and Odo lineages, the core substance of the kata remains remarkably consistent, reflecting the fidelity of its transmission.

The lasting significance of Kakazu no Tekko lies in its representation of the adaptive spirit of postwar Okinawan kobudō. During a time when many weapon traditions faced the risk of being lost to modernization, teachers like Kakazu, Matayoshi, and Odo preserved and elevated the tekko by codifying its principles for teaching, demonstration, and international dissemination. Its endurance across multiple lineages illustrates how a shared respect for combative logic can surpass stylistic boundaries and ensure continuity for future generations.

As a result, practitioners ensure that Kakazu no Tekko is more than just a technical sequence; it serves as a living connection between Okinawa's creativity, its culture of adaptation, and the global practice of kobudō today.

SECTION VIII – TINEBE-JUTSU KATA
Okinawa's Shield: The Art of Cover and Counter

The combination of tinbē (shield) and rochin (short spear) is one of the most distinctive aspects of Okinawan kobudō. Shields could be made from materials such as vine, wood, or even turtle shell, and were paired with a spear about the length of the forearm. This pairing likely reflects both local innovation and influences from Southeast Asia, where similar combinations were commonly used.

In Okinawan martial practices, the tinbē and rochin represent the duality of protection and counterattack, simultaneously deflecting attacks with the shield while thrusting or striking with the spear. Their use in kobudō highlights the Ryukyuan ability to synthesize martial techniques by incorporating local resources and external influences into a unique system. As a cultural artifact, the tinbē-rochin pairing symbolizes balance: defense and offense working together in a cohesive practice.

Kanegawa no Tinbe
Okinawa's Ancestral Shield

Introduction to Kanagawa no Tinbe

Amid the lore of Okinawan kobudō, the tinbe, a humble shield often crafted from turtle shell or cane, evokes images of ancient Ryukyu warriors defending against invaders, yet historical evidence suggests its formal kata, like Kanegawa no Tinbe, emerged not from feudal battles but from 20th-century efforts to preserve eclectic weapon arts amid cultural upheaval, challenging romantic notions of timeless peasant ingenuity. Unlike many kata whose origins are unclear, this particular form is believed to descend from the family line of Taira Shinken, a prominent preservationist of modern kobudō. It is said that he inherited it from his grandfather in Kanagawa. If this lineage is accurate, it represents not just a martial practice but also a rare familial legacy within the broader context of Okinawan weapon arts.

The kata focuses on the paired use of the tinbe (盾, shield) and rochin (短槍, short spear), which is one of the most specialized and least commonly taught combinations in kobudō. Together, these weapons embody a martial strategy distinct from the long-staff and bladed traditions that prevail in Okinawan practice: they enable simultaneous cover and counterattack; compact yet decisive movements.

This chapter will explore the etymology and significance of the kata's name, trace its origins within both family and institutional contexts, analyze the combative principles it encompasses, and follow its transmission through modern lineages. In doing so, it positions Kanegawa no Tinbe not merely as an unusual form within the kobudō curriculum, but as a cultural artifact that intertwines Okinawan ingenuity with a strand of familial memory.

Exploring the Essence of Kanegawa no Tinbe

- **Traditional Notation**: 鐘川のティンベ
- **Script Breakdown**:

    o 鐘川 "Kanegawa" familial surname.

    o の possessive particle—"of".

    o ティンベ "Tinbe" shield; rendered in katakana (native weapon).

- **Core Meaning**: "Kanegawa's Shield"; a tinbe kata inherited from Taira's familial branch.
- **Modern Interpretations**: Understood as a heritage form passed down through Taira's ancestor.
- **Conflicting Ideas & Origins**: Attribution to Taira's grandfather is universally accepted; no real dispute is recorded.

The name Kanegawa no Tinbe (鐘川のティンベ) combines a reference to place and lineage with a designation of the weapon itself. Kanegawa (鐘川) is both a family name and a locality. In this context, most scholars interpret it as denoting the ancestral home of Taira Shinken, whose grandfather is said to have transmitted the form. Tinbe (ティンベ), written in katakana, is the Okinawan term for "shield," likely derived from a southern Chinese martial arts tradition that often used a rattan shield known as tengpai, in combination with a short sword.

Within the records of the Ryukyu Kobudō Hozon Shinkokai, the kata is consistently identified as one "passed down to Taira Shinken from his grandfather," and no competing claims of authorship or alternative naming traditions have gained traction. This stability contrasts with many kobudō kata, whose identities are blurred by overlapping lineages and shifting attributions.

Culturally, the name is significant because it ties a kata not only to a weapon but to a family and a place. By preserving the designation Kanegawa, the kata carries a marker of personal identity and ancestral transmission within its title; an unusual attribute in Okinawan kobudō, where most kata are linked to locations, descriptive images, or legendary figures rather than direct familial heritage. In this sense, the name of Kanegawa no Tinbe embodies both technical continuity and a rare act of cultural memory.

Kanegawa no Tinbe's Historical Roots

The kata Kanegawa no Tinbe occupies a unique position in Okinawan kobudō as a form explicitly linked to family transmission, now practiced by the public. According to lineage accounts, Taira Shinken inherited this kata from his grandfather, incorporating it into his personal martial heritage before it gained wider circulation. Unlike many weapon forms that Taira later codified through collection and reconstruction, this kata represents a direct connection to ancestral practice that he carried into his system.

Its origins predate the upheavals of the 20th century, likely preserved within a familial context where martial skills were maintained alongside daily life. However, its survival can be primarily attributed to Taira's postwar efforts at preservation. In the aftermath of World War II, as Okinawan culture faced both physical devastation and rapid modernization, Taira established the Ryukyu Kobudō Hozon Shinkokai to safeguard endangered weapon traditions. By integrating Kanegawa no Tinbe within this curriculum, he ensured that what had once been a private heritage became part of a collective repertoire accessible to future generations.

The form itself reflects the native combination of shield and short spear, a distinctive Ryukyuan weapon set that has analogues in Southeast Asia but developed in uniquely Okinawan ways. Unlike some of Taira's other codified kata, which drew upon multiple sources, Kanegawa no Tinbe appears to represent a faithful preservation of his grandfather's practice rather than a reconstruction. In this respect, the kata embodies both continuity and resilience: a personal inheritance transformed into a shared cultural legacy.

Applying Kanegawa no Tinbe's Combat Wisdom

At the heart of Kanegawa no Tinbe lies a dynamic interplay between defense and offense, demonstrated through the coordinated use of a shield and a short spear. The kata emphasizes the shield's crucial role as a protective barrier for the torso and head, while the spear delivers sudden thrusts, hooks, and slashes. This creates a rhythm of alternating phases: an opening sequence marked by guarded, defensive movements, followed by a transition into assertive counter-offensives where the rochin takes the initiative.

The stances are compact and functional, designed to enhance balance and mobility in confined or uneven terrain. The yori-ashi (sliding half-step) allows for controlled advances without sacrificing coverage, while the tsuru-dachi (crane stance) supports feints, retreats, and sudden redirections. Bent-knee postures distribute weight evenly, enabling rooted evasion and explosive counterstrikes. Power generation comes from the hips and waist, producing circular, flowing motions that reflect Chinese-influenced body mechanics integrated into Okinawan practice.

The technical repertoire includes shield blocks and parries, thrusts to the midline, inside and outside slashes, and upward strikes that initiate from low positions. The shield is not a passive tool; it obscures the opponent's vision, absorbs incoming force, and creates openings for the rochin to exploit. Hooking actions can destabilize or control an adversary's weapon, while hidden maneuvers, such as feints or concealed thrusts, emphasize the importance of deception.

Bunkai applications consistently highlight close-quarters defense: intercepting an attack with the shield, parrying with the rochin, and countering within the same beat. Internal aspects, such as breath control timed with strikes, rooted stances, and deliberate shifts in body alignment, reinforce the kata's focus on efficiency and protection.

In this way, Kanegawa no Tinbe presents a compact yet sophisticated system of principles, exemplifying the Okinawan ability to adapt their environment, equipment, and body mechanics into an integrated martial logic.

Kanegawa no Tinbe's Evolving Traditions

Since its preservation by Taira Shinken, Kanegawa no Tinbe has been handed down through several of his successor organizations, maintaining its essential structure, while performance details have varied across lineages. Within the Ryukyu Kobujutsu Hozon Shinkokai, founded by Taira and later continued by Inoue Motokatsu, the kata serves as the core transmission of shield-and-spear practice. Eisuke Akamine, Taira's senior student in Okinawa, also safeguarded this form, and his successors, especially Hiroshi Akamine of the Shimbukan, continue to present it as a vital part of their kobudō curriculum. Other branches, such as the Ryukyu Kobudō Tesshinkan under Tamayose Hidemi, include the kata with a specific emphasis on its bunkai, providing students with structured applications alongside performance. Beyond Okinawa, many Taira-affiliated dojos around the world also preserve this form. In recent years, it has been adopted into other systems, including the Matsumura Seito Kenshinkan, where it was formally incorporated by Kise Isao in 2023.

While the framework of the kata remains unified, stylistic distinctions have emerged in the details of execution and interpretation. Some lineages emphasize using the shield for a dropping deflection followed by an immediate spear thrust, while others advocate bracing the tinbe against the body to absorb impact before countering. Head-level defenses also show slight variations: certain schools focus on deflecting with the shield while thrusting around its edge, whereas others prefer more direct parries. Differences in bunkai focus are apparent as well, with some instructors highlighting the shield's trapping capacity, while others emphasize evasive footwork or the rhythm of coordinated counters.

The performance lines (embusen) are generally straightforward, although minor adjustments exist between organizations. Differences in karate backgrounds, such as Shorin-ryu's snap-like chinkuchi or Goju-ryu's emphasis on hard-soft dynamics, can influence how practitioners generate power within the kata. However, these refinements are not reinterpretations; they reflect natural expressions of pedagogical environments and personal training philosophies.

Consequently, Kanegawa no Tinbe provides a shared foundation among Taira's descendants, while simultaneously highlighting the diverse adaptations of Okinawan kobudō according to lineage, instructor, and context. Its shield-based logic, though relatively unique within kobudō curricula, reinforces principles evident in other weapons, such as the tonfa, demonstrating the adaptability of Okinawan martial methods. Unlike many forms that carry folkloric legends, its origin is firmly tied to Taira's own familial inheritance, giving it a notably direct lineage and grounding its place in the living history of Okinawan weapons practice.

Kanegawa no Tinbe's Lasting Impact

Kanegawa no Tinbe is one of the few kobudō kata that can be definitively linked to both familial lineage and institutional preservation. Its name ties it to the Taira family's ancestral home in Kanegawa and highlights the uniquely Okinawan nature of the shield-and-spear combination. Taira Shinken inherited the kata from his grandfather and later codified it through the Ryukyu Kobudō Hozon Shinkokai. This form reflects both private transmission and postwar systematization.

Technically, the kata showcases the practical integration of the shield and spear: it involves blocking and framing with the tinbe while countering with decisive thrusts, slashes, or feints from the rochin. Its structure shifts from defensive control to offensive momentum, teaching adaptability in close-range combat and illustrating the balance between protection and decisiveness central to Okinawan martial strategy. Unlike many weapon forms that have been altered through reinterpretation, Kanegawa no Tinbe has remained relatively stable across generations, a testament to its clarity of design and the reverence with which it is preserved.

Beyond its technical aspects, Kanegawa no Tinbe symbolizes how Okinawan kobudō preserves cultural identity through continuity, even amidst historical upheaval. Preserved by Taira Shinken, who learned it from his grandfather, this kata incorporates Chinese-influenced shield and spear techniques, reflecting Ryukyu's syncretic martial heritage. Its fluid parries, precise stabs, and rooted stances embody practical self-defense strategies suited to the concealed-weapon needs during the Satsuma occupation. Today, Kanegawa no Tinbe resonates in dojos worldwide, perpetuating Taira's legacy of philosophical humility, technical ingenuity, and Ryukyuan resilience against cultural erosion.

Although the early reliance on oral transmission poses challenges, conducting deeper archival research through family records, oral histories, or digitized teaching archives could further illuminate its early development. In an era of global transmission and digital preservation, Kanegawa no Tinbe serves as a living bridge between the past and present, ensuring that Okinawa's essence is honored. At the same time, martial practice adapts to future generations.

Conclusion: Kata as Living Heritage

The kata of Okinawa are not merely sequences of techniques; they are living expressions of memory, carrying the legacy of centuries of Ryukyuan struggle, ingenuity, and resilience. From the quiet exchanges between Chinese envoys and Okinawan scholars to the adaptations made under Satsuma supervision, kata embody an unbroken thread of a culture that has found strength in subtlety and survival in creativity.

For practitioners, kata serve as a discipline for both body and mind. Each stance, strike, and breath recalls lessons first learned in village courtyards and castle grounds, teaching principles of balance, leverage, and timing that remain relevant today, just as they were for the warriors of the past. For historians and cultural enthusiasts, kata provide insights into the dialogue between Okinawa and the wider world: influences from China, Japan, and subtle echoes from Southeast Asian trade networks are evident, yet each form has been uniquely shaped to reflect the needs and identity of Okinawa.

Moreover, kata are not static relics. They have been reinterpreted, restructured, and revitalized by successive generations. Itosu adapted karate for schools, Taira Shinken preserved kobudō from obscurity, and modern teachers have taken these traditions abroad, from Funakoshi Gichin's introduction of karate to mainland Japan in the early 20th century to the establishment of international dojos today. This adaptability is a testament to their vitality: kata endure not by being frozen in time, but by evolving while retaining their core essence.

Looking ahead, the practice of kata offers more than just martial skill; it serves as a bridge across time and culture, connecting us to the values of discipline, humility, and resilience that shaped Okinawa's past. From Sanchin's internal battles to the whirling flails of Matayoshi no Nunchaku, these forms invite ongoing exploration. They also remind practitioners of their responsibility: to study deeply, teach faithfully, and preserve kata not merely as choreography, but as living expressions of a people's history and spirit.

In this way, kata remain what they have always been: a training ground and a time capsule, a discipline and a story, art and heritage. To engage in kata is to step into Okinawa's history and to carry that legacy forward for future generations. As Itosu Anko emphasized in his Ten Precepts, "Karate cannot be quickly learned. Like a slow moving bull, it eventually travels a thousand leagues. If one trains diligently for about three or four hours every day, after three or four years one's body will undergo a great transformation revealing the very essence of karate."

For further reading, consult the bibliography, including Morio Higaonna's "The History of Karate: Okinawan Goju-Ryu" for insights on Higaonna Kanryo and Taira Shinken's "Ryukyu Kobudo Taikan: An Encyclopedia of Ancient Ryukyuan Martial Arts" as compiled in Patrick McCarthy's "Ancient Okinawan Martial Arts: Koryu Uchinadi, Vol. 1."

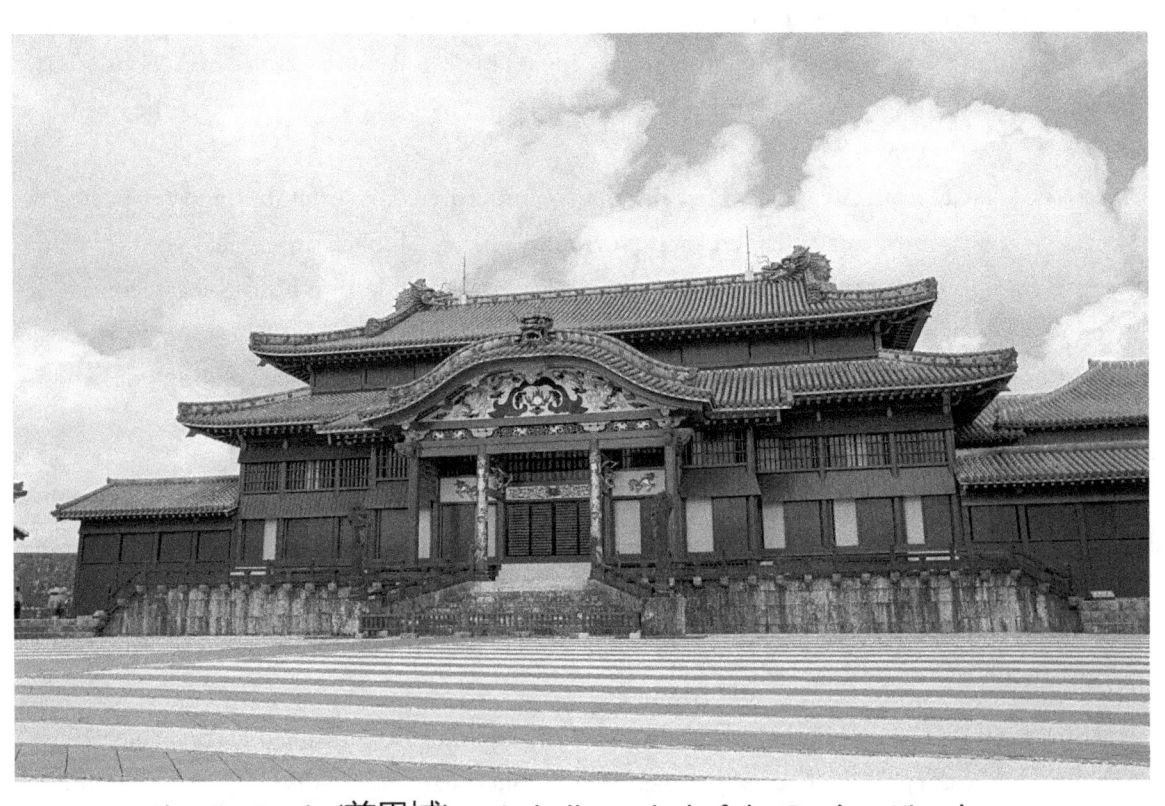

Shurijo Castle (首里城) main hall, symbol of the Ryukyu Kingdom.

(July 2019)

GLOSSARY OF KEY TERMS

Note: This glossary provides definitions of recurring technical, cultural, and historical terms. For the meanings and etymology of individual kata names, see Appendix: Kata Name Etymology. For biographies of historical figures, see Appendix: Key Historical Figures.

A

- Anza (安座) — Cross-legged seated posture, often used for meditation or kata openings.

B

- Bo (棒) — Wooden staff, typically about 6 shaku (~180 cm) in length; primary weapon in Okinawan kobudō.

- Bojutsu (棒術) — Martial art of staff techniques.

- Bunkai (分解) — Application and analysis of kata movements for combat use.

- Bubishi (武備志) — Classical Chinese martial manual preserved in Okinawa; often called the "Bible of Karate."

C

- Chikuden / Chikuden Peichin (筑殿親雲上) — Honorary Yukatchu title or rank sometimes seen in historical records; a formal designation within the pechin class. See also Pechin; Yukatchu.

- Chinkuchi (チンクチ) — Instantaneous muscular contraction and joint alignment used to generate short-range power.

- Chishi (力石) — Traditional Okinawan strength training implement: stone weight on a wooden handle.

- Chudan (中段) — Middle level (torso area); used for strikes/blocks targeting the midsection.

D

- Dachi (立ち) — Stance or posture (e.g., sanchin-dachi, shiko-dachi).
    - Heisoku-dachi (閉足立ち) — "Closed-feet stance"; feet together, heels and toes touching; used for attention or formal bowing.
    - Heiko-dachi (平行立ち) — "Parallel stance"; feet shoulder-width apart, toes pointing forward; relaxed ready stance in some kata.
    - Kiba-dachi (騎馬立ち) — "Horse-riding stance"; feet wide, parallel, knees deeply bent; strong lateral stability, used in some Shorin-ryu and Shotokan kata.
    - Kokutsu-dachi (後屈立ち) — "Back-bent stance" or "rear stance"; weight primarily on the rear leg (~70%), front foot light; used defensively to create distance and absorb force.

- o Musubi-dachi (結び立ち) — "Joined-heel stance"; heels together, toes angled outward ~45°, formal open stance used in bowing/opening sequences.

- o Naihanchi-dachi (内歩進立ち) — Also called Naihanchi shiko-dachi; narrow horse stance with feet turned slightly inward; knees pressing outward for lateral power. Core stance of the Naihanchi kata.

- o Neko-ashi-dachi (猫足立ち) — "Cat-foot stance"; rear-weighted stance (~90% on back leg), front foot light with ball of foot touching; promotes quick evasion.

- o Renoji-dachi (レの字立ち) — "Letter レ stance"; front foot forward, rear foot at 45° forming a shape like the katakana レ; light transitional stance used in some kata.

- o Sanchin-dachi (三戦立ち) — "Three Battles stance"; rooted, inward-tension stance; knees adducted, feet turned slightly inward; central to Naha-te kata for stability and power.

- o Shiko-dachi (四股立ち) — "Sumo-like stance"; wide stance with feet angled outward; knees pushed out, weight evenly distributed; similar to kiba-dachi but toes point outwards.

- o Tsuru-ashi-dachi (鶴足立ち) — "Crane stance"; one-leg stance with the other foot drawn up (varies by kata); used for balance and evasion; also called tsuru-dachi.

- o Zenkutsu-dachi (前屈立ち) — "Forward-bent stance"; long front stance; front knee bent over ankle, rear leg straight; weight forward (~60–70%), used for driving linear techniques.

- Dojo (道場) — Training hall for martial arts practice.

E

- Embusen (演武線) — The "performance line" or floor pattern traced during kata execution; helps visualize combat scenarios.

- Empi (猿臂) — Elbow strike; literally "monkey's elbow."

- Eku (エーク / 櫂) — Okinawan oar weapon used in kobudō.

G

- Gedan (下段) — Lower level (below the belt); targets for low strikes/kicks/blocks.

- Goju-ryu (剛柔流) — "Hard-soft style," Naha-te lineage founded by Miyagi Chojun.

- Gyaku-zuki (逆突き) — Reverse punch delivered with the rear hand.

H

- Hajime (始め) — Command to begin practice or kata.

- Hiza (膝) — Knee; appears in terms like hiza-geri (knee strike).

- Hojo Undo (補助運動) — "Supplemental exercises," traditional Okinawan strength and conditioning drills.

I

- Ibuki (息吹) — Explosive diaphragmatic breathing method, used especially in Naha-te kata.

J

- Jiyu-kumite (自由組手) — Free sparring; non-scripted exchange of techniques.
- Jitte (十手) — Truncheon with side prong; also a kobudō weapon.
- Jodan (上段) — Upper level (head/neck); targets for high strikes/blocks.

K

- Kakete (掛け手) — Hooking hand; technique for grabbing/trapping limbs.
- Kama (鎌) — Traditional sickle; in kobudō, often used in pairs. Originated as a farming tool.
- Ki (気) — Internal energy or life force; cultivated through breath and focus in internal kata like Sanchin.
- Kiai (気合) — Focused shout combining spirit and breath.
- Kihon (基本) — Basic techniques; foundational drills for stances, strikes, blocks.
- Kime (決め) — Focus or decisive tension at technique's end; combines muscular contraction and intent.
- Kobudo (古武道) — "Old martial ways," Okinawan weapons traditions (bo, sai, eku, tonfa, kama, nunchaku, etc.).
- Kumite (組手) — "Meeting of hands," sparring practice.

M

- Mae-geri (前蹴り) — "Front kick"; delivered with the ball of the foot, typically targeting the midsection.
- Mawashi-geri (回し蹴り) — Roundhouse kick.
- Muchimi (ムチミ) — "Sticky/heavy" body feeling; connected, weighted movement principle.

N

- Naha-te (那覇手) — Martial tradition of Naha; precursor to Goju-ryu.
- Nichogama (二丁鎌) — Paired sickles (kama); "nicho" means "two units."
- Nunchaku (ヌンチャク) — Okinawan flail weapon, originally an agricultural implement.

O

- Okinawa-te (沖縄手) — "Okinawan hand," early term for Okinawan martial arts before the term karate was standardized.

P

- Pechin (親雲上) — Mid-ranking member of the Yukatchu (scholar–warrior) class; often served as retainers, palace guards, or martial arts instructors. Frequently appears as an honorific title in historical lineages. See Yukatchu.

- Passai (抜塞) — See Kata Name Etymology Appendix for meaning.

R

- Rochin (ロチン) — Short spear; paired with tinbe in shield-spear kata.

- Rokkishu (六機手) — "Six hand methods" described in the Bubishi; basis for some Naha-te techniques.

- Ryu (流) — "Style" or "school" (e.g., Shorin-ryu, Goju-ryu).

S

- Sai (釵) — Three-pronged truncheon weapon central to Okinawan kobudō.

- Satunushi / Satonushi (里之子) — Lower-ranking Yukatchu title; junior retainers or administrators. See Yukatchu.

- Shorin-ryu (小林流) — "Small/young forest style," Shuri-te and Tomari-te lineage.

- Shuri-te (首里手) — Martial tradition of Shuri; precursor to Shorin-ryu.

T

- Ti / Te (手) — "Hand," early Okinawan term for indigenous martial arts.

- Tinbe (ティンベ) — Shield (often rattan or turtle shell); used defensively with rochin.

- Tonfa (トンファー) — Wooden weapon with side handle, derived from mill handle.

- Tomari-te (泊手) — Martial tradition of the Tomari region; related to Shuri-te and characterized by light, quick movements and unique kata like Wanshu and Chinto.

- Tsuken (津堅) — Small island east of Okinawa's main island; historically associated with notable bo and sai kata (e.g., Tsuken Shitahaku no Sai, Tsuken no Kon).

- Tuite / Tuidi (取手) — Okinawan grappling, joint manipulation, and seizing techniques encoded in kata.

U

- Uchina (ウチナー) — Okinawan word for Okinawa itself; self-referential term by native speakers.

- Uchina-guchi (ウチナー口) — Okinawan language (distinct from standard Japanese); many kata names and historical terms derive from it.

- Uekata (親方) — Senior Yukatchu rank/title; above Pechin; often lords or high officials. See Yukatchu.

- Uechi-ryu (上地流) — Karate style founded by Uechi Kanbun; influenced by Southern Chinese boxing.

- Uke (受け) — Blocking or receiving technique.
  - Gedan-barai (下段払い) — "Low-level sweep"; a downward sweeping block used to deflect attacks to the lower body.
  - Gedan-uke (下段受け) — "Low-level reception/block"; another term for a low block; often used interchangeably with gedan-barai.
  - Jodan-uke (上段受け) — "High-level reception/block"; upward block protecting the head/upper body
  - Kake-uke (掛け受け) — "Hooking block"; circular hooking parry that catches or redirects an opponent's limb.
  -
  - Uchi-uke (内受け) — "Inside block"; inward sweeping middle-level block across the torso.

W

- Waza (技) — Technique or skill.

Y

- Yakusoku-kumite (約束組手) — Pre-arranged sparring drills.
- Yoi (用意) — "Prepare"; command or stance signaling readiness at kata start.
- Yoko-geri (横蹴り) — "Side kick"; lateral kick, often targeting ribs or knees.
- Yukatchu / Yukatcha (良人) — Hereditary Ryukyuan scholar–warrior class. Members were educated in civil administration, Confucian studies, and martial arts; roughly comparable to samurai. Encompasses ranks such as Satunushi, Pechin, Chikuden Peichin, and Uekata.

Z

- Zanshin (残心) — Lingering awareness; mental alertness maintained after a technique or kata.

Appendix: Key Historical Figures of Okinawan Karate and Kobudō

Note: This appendix provides concise biographical notes on notable Okinawan martial arts masters referenced throughout the encyclopedia. Dates are approximate where historical records are incomplete. For deeper lineage discussions, see each kata's chapter and the Lineage/Transmission sections.

Akamine Eisuke (赤嶺栄亮, 1925–1999)
Student of Taira Shinken; founder Ryukyu Kobudō Hozon Shinkokai branch. Led Shimbukan dojo; preserved Taira's kata like Maezato no Tekko.

Annan (安南, dates unknown)
Semi-legendary figure associated with the Chinto kata. Said to have been a shipwrecked Chinese or Vietnamese martial artist who taught indigenous Okinawans. Historical evidence is scant; most references are oral tradition.

Anko Asato (安里安恒, 1827–1906)
Also rendered Azato. A Shuri-te master and mentor of Funakoshi Gichin. Contemporary and colleague of Itosu Anko; emphasized strategy and mental discipline.

Aragaki Seisho (新垣世璋, c. 1840–1920)
Naha/Tomari-te master credited with teaching Unsu, Sochin, and Niseishi. Skilled in weapons and Chinese/Okinawan ceremonial diplomacy.

Chatan Yara (北谷屋良, c. 1658-1756)
Semi-legendary Tomari figure. Credited with Chatan Yara no Sai and Chatan Yara no Kon. Represents early synthesis of Chinese and Okinawan methods.

Chi'kin Kraka / Chikin Chojun / Tsuken Mantaka (知花朝順?, 19th century)
Associated with Chikin Bo. Likely an Okinawan practitioner from Chibana/Chikin region. Historical details scarce; preserved mainly through kata attribution.

Funakoshi Gichin (船越義珍, 1868–1957)
Student of Itosu and Asato; introduced Okinawan karate to mainland Japan. Founded Shotokan; systematized curriculum and adapted kata names.

Higa Peichin (比嘉親雲上, c. 1663-1738)
Shuri-based bushi of the Pechin class. Credited with Higa-related kobudō kata (e.g., Hama Higa no Sai). May have been an ancestor to later Higa karate families; historical data limited.

Higaonna Kanryo (東恩納寛量, 1853–1915)
Naha-te master, studied in Fujian. Brought back Sanchin and related forms; teacher of Miyagi Chojun.

265

Inoue Motokatsu (井上元勝, 1918–1993)

Student of Taira Shinken; founder Ryukyu Kobujutsu Hozonkai. Grandson of PM Katsura Taro; integrated kobudō with karate.

Itosu Anko (糸洲安恒, 1831–1915)

Shuri-te innovator; created Pinan series; introduced karate to public schools.

Kakazu Mitsuo (嘉数光男, dates uncertain, mid-20th c.)

Student of Matayoshi Shinko; creator Kakazu no Tekko. Teacher of Odo Seikichi; postwar kobudō innovator.

Kise Fusei (喜瀬普請, 1935–Present)

Founder of Kenshinkan/OSMKKF. Senior student of Soken Hohan; preserved Matsumura Seito karate and kobudō. Oversaw international spread of his family's tradition.

Kise Isao (喜瀬 功, 1957–2025)

Son of Kise Fusei and heir to the OSMKKF and Kenshinkan traditions. Studied with Hohan Sōken, Kise Fusei, and Yoshio Kuba (Gōjū-ryū). Guided and further codified both Matsumura Seito and Kenshinkan traditions, overseeing grading, instruction, and international growth. Father and teacher of Kise Chōfu; remembered for his humility, discipline, and stewardship of the family's legacy.

Kinjo Hiroshi (金城裕, 1919–2013)

Karate historian; documented kata origins and technical terminology. Practitioner and researcher bridging Okinawan and Japanese karate.

Komesu Ushi (米須牛, 1854-1920)

Student of Chi'kin Kraka, credited with teaching Soken Hohan Kobudō, specifically the kata Chi'kin Bo; historical verification limited to oral tradition.

Kusanku (公相君 / Kusanku, c. 1670-1760)

Chinese envoy and martial artist sent to Ryukyu. Demonstrated Chinese boxing; Kusanku kata named after him. Key link for Chinese influence in Okinawan arts.

Kyan Chotoku (喜屋武朝徳, 1870–1945)

Shuri/Tomari master; transmitted Wanshu, Ananku, Passai, etc. Student of multiple teachers including Matsumura and Matsumora.

Matayoshi Shinko (又吉眞光, 1888–1947)

Founder Matayoshi Kobudō; studied in China. Teacher of Kakazu Mitsuo, and son Matayoshi Shinpo; integrated weapons like kama, nunchaku.

Matayoshi Shinpo (又吉眞豊, 1921–1997)

Son of Shinko; formalized Matayoshi Kobudō Kodokan. Spread kobudō globally; created kata like Matayoshi no Nunchaku.

Matsu Higa (松比嘉, 1790-1870)

One of the first to codify a system of kata and techniques, Matsu Higa was Peichin of Hama Higa island. Believe to have been a student of the Chinese emissaries Zhang Xue Li and later Wanshu, there are several Kobudō kata associated with him.

Matsumora Kosaku (松茂良興作, 1829–1898)

Tomari master; taught Wanshu, Chinto; known for light-footed evasive tactics.

Matsumura Sokon (松村宗棍, 1809–1899)

Seminal Shuri-te master; royal bodyguard; credited with transmitting many foundational kata.

Miyagi Chojun (宮城長順, 1888–1953)

Student of Higaonna; founder of Goju-ryu. Named style "hard-soft."

Motobu Choki (本部朝基, 1870–1944)

Pragmatic fighter; emphasized Naihanchi and kumite. Noted for real combat ability.

Motobu Choyu (本部朝勇, 1857–1927)

Senior Motobu brother; keeper of Motobu Udun-di (palace hand) traditions.

Nagamine Shoshin (長嶺将真, 1907–1997)

Founder Matsubayashi Shorin-ryu; created Fukyugata Ichi; historian of Okinawan masters.

Odo Seikichi (小渡誠吉, 1926–2002)

Founder Okinawa Kenpo Karate Kobudō; student of Kakazu, Matayoshi. Renamed kata like Kakazu no Tekko to Odo no Tekkos Ni.

Sakugawa Kanga / Kangi (佐久川寛賀, 1733–1815)

"Tode" Sakugawa; pioneer of bojutsu; teacher of Matsumura. Sakugawa no Kon bears his name.

Soken Hohan (祖堅方範, 1889–1982)

Grandson of Nabe Matsumura; 20th-century head of Matsumura Seito Shorin-ryu. Teacher of Kise Fusei.

Taira Shinken (平信賢, 1897–1970)

Born Maezato Shinken; founder Ryukyu Kobudō Hozon Shinkokai. Codified kata like Maezato no Tekko, Kanegawa no Tinbe; preserved 40+ forms.

Tamayose Hidemi (玉寄秀美, 1949–)

Founder Ryukyu Kobudō Tesshinkan; student of Akamine Eisuke. Preserves Taira lineage; emphasizes bunkai in kata like Maezato no Tekko.

Tawada Shinboku (多和田真睦, 1814–1884)

Okinawan bo/sai expert. Tawada no Sai/Bo named after him.

Tokumine Pechin (徳嶺親雲上, 19th century)

Renowned bo master; exiled after an altercation; Tokumine no Kon attributed to him.

Tsuken Shitahaku (津堅下迫, 1645-1725)

Associated with Tsuken Shitahaku no Sai. Likely kobudō teacher from Tsuken island; primarily preserved through oral lineage.

Uechi Kanbun (上地完文, 1877–1948)

Founder Uechi-ryu; studied Pangai-noon in China. His son Kanei formalized the curriculum.

Wang Ji (汪輯 / Wanshu, c. 1630–1700)

Chinese envoy to Ryukyu; Wanshu kata named after him. Representative of early Chinese influence.

Yonamine Chiru (与那嶺チル, semi-legendary)

Female bushi figure; sometimes associated with Seisan. Likely folklore; symbolic of Okinawan warrior women. Matsumura Sokon's wife.

BIBLIOGRAPHY AND SUGGESTED READING

- Bishop, M. D. (2000). Okinawan Weaponry: Hidden Methods, Ancient Myths of Kobudo & Te. Tuttle Publishing. (Covers the historical myths and methods behind Okinawan weapons like tonfa, nunchaku, and kama, with insights into kata origins.)

- Bishop, M. D. (2017). Zen Odyssey: An Okinawan Karate & Martial Arts Journey. Lulu.com. (A personal exploration of Okinawan karate history, including kata development and Ryukyuan cultural context.)

- Funakoshi, G. (1935/2001). Karate-do Kyohan: The Master Text (O. Tsutomu, Trans.). Kodansha International. (Foundational text on karate principles, with discussions of kata like those adapted from Okinawan origins for Japanese schools.)

- Funakoshi, G. (2003). The Twenty Guiding Principles of Karate: The Spiritual Legacy of the Master (J. Teramoto, Trans.). Kodansha International. (Philosophical insights into karate's mindset, relevant to the internal principles in foundational kata like Sanchin.)

- Guarelli, A. (2016). Okinawan Kobudo: The History, Tools, and Techniques of the Ancient Martial Art. Skyhorse Publishing. (Detailed history and techniques for kobudo weapons, including kata for bo, sai, tonfa, and more, with Matayoshi lineage focus.)

- Higaonna, M. (2001). The History of Karate: Okinawan Goju-ryu. Dragon Books. (Comprehensive history of Naha-te styles, emphasizing Sanchin and its Chinese roots via Higaonna Kanryo.)

- Hopkins, G. (2020). Wandering Along the Way of Okinawan Karate: Contemplations on Goju-ryu. North Atlantic Books. (Philosophical and historical reflections on Goju-ryu kata, including Seisan, Suparinpei, and breathing techniques.)

- Inoue, M. (1972–1974). Ryukyu Kobujutsu (Vols. 1–3). (Rare printed series on traditional kobudo kata, including sai forms like those attributed to Chatan Yara and Tsuken Shitahaku.)

- Kane, L. A., & Wilder, K. (2005). The Way of Kata: A Comprehensive Guide to Deciphering Martial Applications. YMAA Publication Center. (Practical bunkai for Okinawan kata, applicable to intermediate and advanced forms like Passai and Kusanku.)

- Kim, R. (1982). Kobudo: Okinawan weapons of Matsu Higa, Hama Higa, and Chatan Yara (Vols. 1–3). Unique Publications. (Illustrated guides to specific kobudo kata for sai, tonfa, and kama, with historical attributions.)

- Marshall, S. R. (2019). Okinawan Kobudo: A History of Weaponry Styles and Masters. Independently published. (Overview of kobudo masters like Taira Shinken and weapon-specific kata histories.)

- McCarthy, P. (1995). Bubishi: The Bible of Karate. Tuttle Publishing. (Translated ancient text on karate's Chinese origins, vital for understanding foundational principles in kata like Naihanchi and Seisan.)
- McCarthy, P. (1987). Classical Kata of Okinawan Karate. Ohara Publications. (Detailed breakdowns of Shorin-ryu and other Okinawan kata, including origins, techniques, and patriarchs.)
- Nishiuchi, I. (2000). The Best of Okinawan Martial Arts Weapons Series. (Multi-volume set on nunchaku, tonfa, and other weapons, with kata demonstrations and history.)
- Quast, A. (2015). A Stroll Along Ryukyu Martial Arts History. Independently published. (Chronological history of Ryukyu martial arts, covering kata evolutions and influences from China and Japan.)

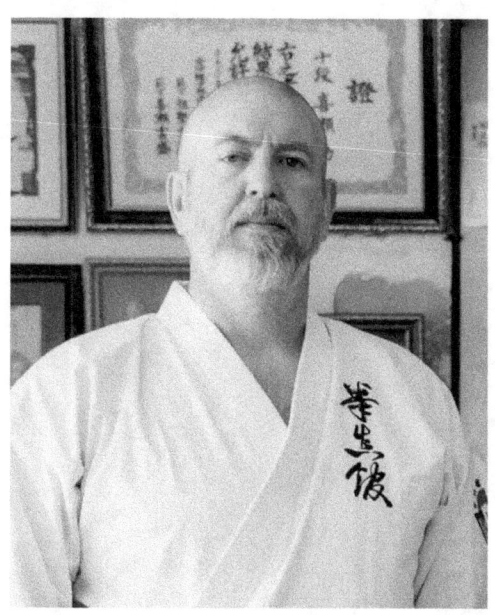

ABOUT THE AUTHOR

Nathan Batson has dedicated nearly forty years to exploring and teaching the martial traditions of Okinawa. As both a lifelong practitioner and researcher, he combines hands-on training with historical study, making karate, kobudō, and tuite accessible to practitioners and curious readers alike.

He is the founder of the Tyler Karate Academy, where he has taught thousands of students and led seminars across the United States and abroad. His training includes senior ranks in karate, kobudō, and tuite, with additional study in Musō Jikiden Eishin-ryū iaidō, Filipino martial arts, judo, and jiu-jitsu.

Nathan is the author of the *Okinawa Kata Encyclopedia: Exploring Ryukyu's Hidden Secrets*, a comprehensive reference work documenting the history, lineage, and practice of Okinawan karate and kobudō kata. His forthcoming work, *Foundations of Okinawan Tuite: Building a Path to Mastery*, explores the often-overlooked principles of Okinawa's grappling arts. Inspired by his students and shaped by research trips to Okinawa, he writes to preserve and share the enduring spirit of Uchinā Damashī, the Okinawan spirit that defines both culture and martial soul.